Guidelines
for
Perinatal Care

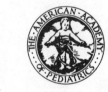

American Academy of Pediatrics

The American College
of Obstetricians and Gynecologists

Supported in part by
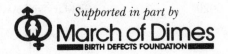
March of Dimes
BIRTH DEFECTS FOUNDATION

Design: Michael Dodd
Cover Art: Marilyn Kaufman

Guidelines for Perinatal Care was developed through the cooperative efforts of the AAP Committee on Fetus and Newborn and the ACOG Committee on Obstetrics: Maternal and Fetal Medicine. The guidelines should not be viewed as a body of rigid rules. They are general and intended to be adapted to many different situations, taking into account the needs and resources particular to the locality, the institution, or type of practice. Variations and innovations that demonstrably improve the quality of patient care are to be encouraged rather than restricted. The purpose of these guidelines will be well served if they provide a firm basis on which local norms may be built. The segments related to obstetric practice do not replace the ACOG *Standards for Obstetric-Gynecologic Services,* but expand on the principles suggested in the ACOG manual.

Library of Congress Catalog Card Number: 83-71148
ISBN: 0-910761-04-3

Quantity prices available on request. Address all inquiries to either:

American Academy of Pediatrics
P.O. Box 1034
Evanston, Illinois 60204

American College of Obstetricians
   and Gynecologists
600 Maryland Avenue, SW, Suite
   300 East
Washington, DC 20024

Editorial Committee

Editors:	Alfred W. Brann Jr., MD, FAAP
	Robert C. Cefalo, MD, PhD, FACOG
Associate Editors:	Fredric D. Frigoletto, MD, FACOG
	George A. Little, MD, FAAP
Managing Editor:	Rebecca D. Rinehart
Staff:	Jean D. Lockhart, MD, AAP
	Ervin E. Nichols, MD, ACOG
	Shirley A. Shelton, ACOG

AAP Committee on Fetus and Newborn

Current Members,
1982–1983:

George A. Little, MD *(Chairman, 1981–present)*
Rita G. Harper, MD
Louis I. Levy, MD
M. Jeffrey Maisels, MD
Gerald Merenstein, MD, Col,
 MC
Ronald L. Poland, MD
Philip G. Rhodes, MD
Philip Sunshine, MD

Liaison Representatives
James R. Allen, MD, MPH
Paula Brill, MD
Alfred A. deLorimier, MD
Fredric D. Frigoletto, MD
Dennis Hey, DO
V. Robert Kelly, MD
Gerard Ostheimer, MD
Eugene Outerbridge, MD
George J. Peckham, MD

ACOG Committee on Obstetrics: Maternal and Fetal Medicine

Contributors and Consultants

The chapters in this manual have no specific authors; members from the two committees were responsible for preparing initial drafts of chapters or sections. Subsequently, after much committee deliberation and consideration, opinions of all individuals involved—both contributors and consultants—were integrated in chapters and then further reviewed, modified, and refined by the editorial committee. The work of individual AAP/ACOG committee members and the following contributors and consultants was essential to the evolution of the professional recommendations reflected in *Guidelines for Perinatal Care*.

Garland Anderson, MD
Thomas Barden, MD
John Barton, MD
Richard Baum, MD
Lillian Blackmon, MD
Drusilla Burnham, PhD
L. Joseph Butterfield, MD
Janet Collins, MSW
Carlyle Crenshaw, MD
Preston Dilts, MD
John Fishburne, MD
Roger Freeman, MD
William Fuller, MD
Steven Gabbe, MD
Sprague Gardiner, MD
Charles E. Gibbs, MD
Ronald Gibbs, MD
Anita Glicken, MSW
C.P. Goplerud, MD
Perry Henderson, MD
Peter Honeyfield, MD
Vince Hutchins, MD
L. Stanley James, MD
Harold Kaminetzky, MD
Linda Krell, MD
Rosanna Lenker, CNM
Lula Lubchenco, MD

Jerold F. Lucey, MD
Brian McCarthy, MD
Donald McNellis, MD
Frederick Meier, MD
Frank Miller, MD
Gilles Monif, MD
Sr. Alice Montgomery, RN
James Morrison, MD
Andre J. Nahmias, MD
William O'Brien, MD
Joan C. Offutt, MPA
William Oh, MD
Roy Pitkin, MD
Paul Placek, PhD
Ruth Redman, RN
C. Thomas Reynold, MD
Roger Roghat, MD
George Ryan Jr., MD
Ben Sachs, MD
Arthur Salisbury, MD
Harold Schulman, MD
Charles R. Scriver, MD
Sr. Mary Stella Simpson, CNM
Philip Sumner, MD
James M. Sutherland, MD
Reginald Tsang, MD
Berry Vohr, MD

These guidelines are dedicated to Sprague H. Gardiner, MD, FACOG, Chairman of the original Committee on Perinatal Health, and L. Joseph Butterfield, Director, Office of Regional Program Development at Children's Hospital, Denver, Colorado.

This monograph is here dedicated to ... ... Gardner, MD, FACOG, Chairman of ... ... of Health, and ... ... Director, Office of Regional Program Development at ... Bureau of Hygiene, Dar es Salaam, ...

Contents

3 Personnel for Perinatal Services 37

4 Perinatal Care Services 47

5 Maternal and Neonatal Follow-Up Care

Foreword

Early efforts to enhance perinatal care focused on evaluating maternal and neonatal services within a region, assessing needs, and developing a system designed to increase the accessibility of care, particularly for high-risk mothers and infants.

Regionalization was still a relatively new concept in 1977 when the sixth edition of *Standards and Recommendations for Hospital Care of Newborn Infants* was published by the American Academy of Pediatrics. That publication gave detailed recommendations for the level of services an institution provided, emphasizing the need to make the most skilled, intense care available to the mothers and infants at highest risk.

It has become increasingly apparent to those involved with the evolution of regionalization that further progress in improving maternal and infant care requires a coordinated approach to perinatal care, from conception through the postpartum and neonatal periods. Perinatal care has emerged as a concept that, by improving the professional, educational, and service capabilities of perinatal care programs, has united obstetric and pediatric efforts toward the common goal of improved care for mothers and infants.

The American Academy of Pediatrics and The American College of Obstetricians and Gynecologists, both of which have considerable backgrounds in promulgating guidelines of care, share this common objective. In the mid-1970s, representatives from both organizations served on the March of Dimes Committee on Perinatal Health that developed *Toward Improving the Outcome of Pregnancy,* which defined resources essential for the provision of specific services. This served as the impetus for further unified efforts directed toward lowering maternal and infant morbidity and mortality.

As a result, the first of what was to become an annual event—a joint meeting of the ACOG Committee on Obstetrics: Maternal and Fetal Medicine and the AAP Committee on Fetus and Newborn—took place later that year on November 16, 1978. It was at this meeting that the idea of a perinatal manual was first discussed. It was supported and encouraged by the officers of both organizations, and work on the joint manual began in the Spring of 1980. As it progressed, it became clear that more was happening than joint authorship of a publication; two disciplines were getting to know each other's per-

spectives, problems, and successes, stimulating each other to new
approaches to improving the care of mothers and infants.

This insight, as well as the committee members' combined expertise and diverse backgrounds, is reflected in the first edition of *Guidelines for Perinatal Care,* a new tradition that will surely be followed by
succeeding editions. As with all manuals, the comments, criticisms, and
suggestions received from users will be of enormous help to the committees as they continue their collective effort to improve perinatal
care.

Jean D. Lockhart, MD   Ervin E. Nichols, MD
AAP   ACOG

Preface

Guidelines for Perinatal Care is unique—it exemplifies the cooperative efforts of two disciplines dedicated to the improvement of pregnancy outcome.

Since the beginning of this century, there has been a significant improvement in pregnancy outcome. Initially, during the first 60 years, largely independent and isolated obstetric and pediatric efforts resulted in decreases in the rates of maternal and neonatal mortality. However, with the growing realization that pregnancy outcome can be improved most effectively by integrating the skills and knowledge of multiple disciplines, current collaborative efforts are focusing on the continued reduction of perinatal mortality as well as decreased neonatal morbidity. This multidisciplinary effort has had an impact on perinatal care in three very important areas: improved and expanded understanding of physiology and pathophysiology of the pregnant woman, fetus, and neonate; improved health care delivery through risk assessment and regionalization; and better appreciation of the human childbirth experience and the role of the family.

These concepts have been integrated in *Guidelines for Perinatal Care,* produced through the joint efforts of the American Academy of Pediatrics and The American College of Obstetricians and Gynecologists. The most current factual information, scientific opinions, and practices have been collected and reviewed to formulate this manual, which is intended to set guidelines, not strict operating rules, for providing perinatal care. A deliberate attempt has been made to integrate the concept of family-centered care into every phase of perinatal services and to recommend ideal but attainable objectives. It must be emphasized that increased investment of community resources is essential to the achievement of these objectives and the ultimate goal of optimal contemporary perinatal care. Everyone benefits from improved perinatal services because everyone uses these services at least once in their life.

Guidelines for Perinatal Care incorporates and replaces *Standards and Recommendations for Hospital Care of Newborn Infants,* which has been revised through six editions since its initial publication in 1948 by the AAP Committee on Fetus and Newborn. Each Chapter has been written, reviewed, and edited by members of both the AAP Committee on Fetus and Newborn and the ACOG Committee on

Obstetrics: Maternal and Fetal Medicine. It is designed for use by personnel who provide care to pregnant women, their fetuses, and neonates in both community hospitals and medical centers.

Readers of this manual represent a cross-section of different disciplines within the perinatal community; the intermingling of basic and sophisticated information is necessary to address this diverse audience. Local circumstances must dictate the way in which these guidelines are best interpreted to meet the needs of the particular hospital, community, and system the perinatal unit serves.

Guidelines and recommendations in this manual should be used to form the basis of codes and regulations governing the building and operation of perinatal facilities in many cities and states. It is *not* the intention of this manual to set regulations so rigid as to obstruct responsible attempts at innovation or incorporation of new information into perinatal care practices and the construction of new perinatal units.

The editors and the members of the Committee wish to thank their colleagues and consultants and the administrative staff of both professional societies for their role in developing the first edition of *Guidelines for Perinatal Care*. The continued support and encouragement of both parent Executive Boards have made this a unique privilege. It is hoped that this manual establishes a precedent for the continued improvement of pregnancy outcome.

—Editorial Committee

Introduction

Toward Improving the Outcome of Pregnancy: Recommendations for the Regional Development of Maternal and Perinatal Services was published in 1976 by the March of Dimes. Its purpose was to define the principle of regionalized perinatal care and, in broad and general concepts, to illustrate the approach to developing a system of shared responsibility in providing perinatal services.

The publication was avidly received by most health professionals and planners. Although misinterpretation of the "guidelines and recommendations" as absolutes has at times impeded progress in improving perinatal care and services, the groups involved with the effort to elucidate the concept of regionalization in *Toward Improving the Outcome of Pregnancy* are proud to be associated with its evolution.

In recent years, it has become apparent that there was a need for detailed and specific, up-to-date recommendations for the management of both normal and high-risk patients in the prenatal, perinatal, and neonatal periods. The American Academy of Pediatrics and The American College of Obstetricians and Gynecologists have met this need with the publication of *Guidelines for Perinatal Care*. The two organizations are to be especially thanked and congratulated for having worked jointly to produce this statement of consensus on the optimal management of pregnancy for the mother, fetus, and infant.

The March of Dimes has appropriately recognized its continuing partnership with the Academy and the College by helping to defray the costs of publication and distribution of *Guidelines for Perinatal Care*. We will continue to extend our efforts to implement these guidelines and to give every baby a healthy start in life.

Arthur J. Salisbury, MD, MPH
Vice President for Medical Services
March of Dimes Birth Defects Foundation

chapter 1

Organization of Perinatal Health Care

Regional delivery of perinatal health care is a systems approach in which program components in a geographic area are defined and coordinated. Successful systems meet local needs and support individual physician-patient relationships. They emphasize communication and education, consultation and professional competence in the utilization of services according to patient needs, and cost-effective services, including consolidation when indicated. National and international models for the delivery of perinatal health care on a regional basis have significantly reduced perinatal mortality and morbidity through application of present day knowledge. A systematic approach to perinatal care can reduce perinatal death rates proportionately for both middle and low socioeconomic classes.

The perinatal mortality rate in the under-1500 g birth-weight group clearly demonstrates that regional approaches to newborn care have been effective in the United States. The improvement in the birth-weight-specific neonatal mortality rate of the past two decades appears to be related to the advent of special care for newborns and improved intrapartum management. Although outcome is not necessarily influenced by facility size or number of deliveries per year, the availability of obstetric and pediatric specialists has played an important role in managing low-birth-weight infants and reducing intrapartum asphyxia. For neonates who require intensive care, the benefits of transport have been shown to outweigh the risks when outcomes are compared with those of neonates kept at facilities unable to provide such care.

Studies from the United States, Norway, and Sweden have shown that early diagnosis of prenatal problems, care, and transfer, when indicated, are beneficial to the fetus. Recent evidence suggests that maternal-fetal transport to ensure newborn intensive care at birth further improves neonatal outcome. Morbidity of low-birth-weight neonates, including but not limited to those with respiratory distress syndrome (RDS), is decreased with maternal-fetal transport. In addition, maternal-fetal transport is more economical, both financially and in terms of personnel, than neonatal transport, and it encourages early maternal-neonatal bonding and attachment. Studies have shown the cost of maternal-fetal hospitalization for planned deliveries to be less than the expense of neonatal intensive care when maternal-fetal transport is not utilized, largely because the length of neonatal hospital stay is decreased when maternal-fetal transport is used.

HISTORICAL BACKGROUND

Maternal Mortality

In the United States, maternal mortality had decreased to a level of 6.9/100,000 live births by 1980. There are several reasons for this decline. Significant improvement began years ago when medical or obstetric and gynecologic societies formed committees to review maternal deaths. They defined preventable events; scrutinized maternal and perinatal deaths according to county, state, and national health authorities, as well as professionals; and established open lines of communication. Following this came the development of education and service projects directed toward optimal outcome for the mother, fetus, and neonate. This led to a positive relationship in some localities between professional groups and maternal and child health government agencies and served as a model for other specialties and agencies.

Premature Centers

In the 1920s and 1930s, centers designed to care for premature neonates appeared in the United States, fostered in part by the work of Julius Hess in Chicago. Such units trace some of their origins to the influence of Martin Couney, who organized public exhibitions of small babies at fairs and expositions in Europe and the United States at the turn of the century. While criticized for their commercial motivation, the displays attracted medical attention, including that of Hess. By the 1940s and 1950s, a uniform standard of care based on isolation, thermal stability, nutrition, and specialized nursing care had been established at several locations, and academic perinatal study was under way.

The establishment of these centers was followed by the establishment of neonatal intensive care units at several locations in the 1950s and 1960s, when the intensive care concept was developing in both adult and pediatric medicine. In fact, early descriptions included discussions of neonatal intensive care in conjunction with adult intensive care. During the 1960s, the scope of neonatal care expanded rapidly, resulting in more aggressive medical and surgical care of all neonates; the basic population served remained the low-birth-weight neonate, however. The close relationship between neonatal intensive care and the main body of obstetric practice began to emerge late in the 1960s, although basic concern and preparation for interaction were evident much earlier.

Maternal-Fetal Assessment

The increasing ability to assess both maternal and fetal risks ushered in a new era in obstetric care in the late 1960s and early 1970s. Special knowledge and skills advanced maternal care, while interventions for fetal health, including maturity studies that allow consideration of selective preterm delivery, became a clinical reality. Dialogue between obstetricians and pediatricians became a requirement, not a courtesy, as the parallel development of obstetric and neonatal intensive care resulted in joint centers.

Role of Organizations

Perinatal regionalization systems have been greatly influenced by professional organizations. The American College of Obstetricians and Gynecologists surveyed obstetric practices in the United States in 1967 and defined several problem areas, such as the underutilization of beds, the difficulty encountered by small obstetric services in handling emergency procedures, and deficiencies in the immediate care of the neonate. In 1973, the College stated that one of its goals was to reduce the perinatal mortality rate in the United States to 10/1000 births within 10 years. There was further College emphasis on regional education programs and the development of guidelines for a regional perinatal care system. In 1971, a joint committee of the Society of Obstetricians and Gynaecologists of Canada and the Canadian Paediatric Society, as well as the American Medical Association, took positions in favor of regionalization of perinatal health care.

In 1973, The National Foundation-March of Dimes provided financial and administrative support for the ad hoc Committee on Perinatal Health, an interprofessional and multidisciplinary group representing the American Academy of Family Physicians, the American Academy of Pediatrics, The American College of Obstetricians and Gynecologists, and the American Medical Association. Guidelines for a regional perinatal care system were developed with consultants from other health professions, government agencies, and consumers. The subsequent adoption of these guidelines (published in the report, *Toward Improving the Outcome of Pregnancy*), in principle or with little conceptual modification, by the federal government and over 50% of state legislatures, is evidence of their importance, validity, and timeliness.

The realization that the burgeoning knowledge and care requirements of perinatology mandated special attention led to establishment in the 1970s of the Sub-board of Neonatal-Perinatal Medicine by the American Board of Pediatrics and the Division of Maternal-Fetal Medicine of the American Board of Obstetrics and Gynecology.

THE CONCEPT OF LEVELS AND PROGRAM DEVELOPMENT

A level can be defined as part of the activity of a comprehensive perinatal care system. In *Toward Improving the Outcome of Pregnancy*, the three-level system that has penetrated most existing regional programs and health planning activities is discussed (Table 1–1).

In the past, definitions of levels have tended to emphasize individual hospital care more than the other activities within a regional program. Hospitals with level I programs generally provide services for uncomplicated deliveries and normal neonates. These hospitals tend to be in sparsely populated areas where the number of births is small. Professionals at these units must be able to identify risks as well as manage a mother, fetus, or newborn who unexpectedly may develop life-threatening problems until the patient can be transferred. In hospitals with level II programs services are provided for routine deliveries and normal neonates, as well as for selected high-risk problems of pregnant women and for certain neonatal illnesses. Hospitals with level III programs provide all types of perinatal care, including obstetric and neonatal intensive care, as well as a broad range of subspecialty consultative services. They have been, and will continue to be, located principally at academic institutions, owing to the complexity of the clinical, educational, and research services provided.

Through the conceptual process, levels have been defined to indicate relative areas of responsibility in a comprehensive system of patient care, continuing education, and evaluation. All patients should have access to care at an appropriate level, according to need and regardless

Table 1-1. *Levels of Program Development (I, II, III)*

Levels of basic perinatal network	Activity	Locations	Usual physician leadership
I	Usual focus of patient entry into system Risk assessment Uncomplicated perinatal care Stabilization of unexpected problems Data collection Sponsor of local education	Community hospital or colocated at level II or level III facility	Primary care physician or specialist
II	Level I activities, plus: Diagnosis and treatment of selected high-risk pregnancies and neonatal problems Patient transport Education efforts for part of network	Large community hospitals with many support services or colocated at level III facility	Specialist or subspecialist
III	Usually level I and level II activities,* plus: Diagnosis and treatment of most perinatal problems Research and outcome surveillance Regional education Regional administration	Large medical centers with comprehensive academic programs	Subspecialist

*Some level III facilities, such as level III neonatal units in children's hospitals, many not provide level I and level II services. Regional Resource Centers provide specialized knowledge and skills in academic medical centers (level III) at a subspecialty (academic) level.

of financial status. In most instances, this access and identification within the system is through a personal physician, such as an obstetrician, pediatrician, or family practitioner.

In the future, the concept of three levels will continue to be useful, but program development, as well as patient care, should be incorporated into the definitions. Program development is a dynamic process of regionally identifying needs, allocating resources, initiating activity, evaluating outcome, and then maintaining and adjusting performance. Each institution within a system should go through this process and define its level or sphere of activity within a region. A focus on program development allows for flexibility in the definition of levels and should reflect documented needs and resources.

A regional program is a network coordinating professional services and institutional resources. Each program level is interrelated with others in the regional system. Interrelatedness means no unit can be free-standing. An appropriate forum, such as a regional council, committee, or planning agency that cooperates with professional groups, government or private agencies, and patient advocates, may influence the local structure; however, regional plans that restrict communication or excessively structure or codify levels limit flexibility. Conversely, excessive emphasis on the development of a particular level, especially levels II or III, may prove detrimental. Varying levels of care can be provided concurrently in level II or III units. Under certain circumstances, children's hospitals may provide neonatal care without direct involvement with a specific obstetric service. However, such children's hospital units should be part of a total perinatal system. The emphasis must be on optimal care of the perinatal patient.

In each region, levels of program development can and should be categorized, either for the entire spectrum of perinatal care or, initially, for part of the total system, such as neonatal care (appendix A is a representative categorization). Although manuals or information from other regions can serve as a base for categorization, working groups from individual regions should ensure that the final product is appropriate for their own region.

Owing to the highly specialized and costly resources involved, regional resource centers should be considered to provide leadership, knowledge, and special skills for each network. These cooperative efforts should be directed toward cost-effective management of specific specialized problems.

Accountability for all levels of program development should be considered in regional planning, although mechanisms of accountability that are based on factors such as patient access, quality assurance of individual practice standards, and supervision of program direction have yet to be well defined for regional programs. A regional council might be given this responsibility. These councils should have both professional and nonprofessional members, and may include a representative of a state government unit such as the Bureau of Maternal and Child Health.

In a flexible system based on levels of program development, hospital leaders have the opportunity and obligation to help determine their hospitals' roles within a broad regional context. Totally independent activity of an institution without consideration of all factors is inappropriate and may obstruct the attainment of regional goals and objectives. Completely independent delineation of program involvement has led to centralization in some locations. Conversely, the concept of flexibility in program development does not justify the proliferation of multiple small units unless such a system is part of a regional plan and clearly in the best interest of patient care and efficient use of resources.

GOALS AND OBJECTIVES

An organized perinatal care program must be based on goals and objectives directed at the entire perinatal population. Service, education, and research must be balanced to allow for increasingly better care through expansion of professional knowledge and skills, proper allocation of resources, and outcome evaluation. In this manner, all health care providers and consumers are considered.

Broad goals for national and regional perinatal programs include (1) the reduction of maternal, fetal, and neonatal mortality and morbidity to the lowest attainable levels; and (2) efficient utilization of available resources, balanced with patient needs. Health care needs and morbidity rates should be broadly interpreted to include psychosocial as well as physical or organic problems. The concept of an irreducible minimum in mortality or morbidity rates is unacceptable as a limit to improvement in perinatal medicine.

National objectives should serve as guidelines for regions, but they should be individualized to meet local needs. The problems and resources of one region may be quite different from those of other regions or those of the nation as a whole. Rural and economically deprived areas may require special consideration, for example. State or regional planning agencies are justified in altering national recommendations after they have assessed local needs and resources.

Objectives determined by each region should be implemented for a reasonable but defined length of time, then reevaluated and revised periodically.

Efforts to attain objectives are most effective if the service, education, and evaluation aspects of the total system are taken into account. For example, state or regional groups planning to provide intermediate level nursery services should consider the technical nature of the services needed, the ongoing educational needs of the personnel who are to deliver services, and the means of evaluating outcome. A process that limits attention to allocation of service needs, such as beds, and does not allow for consideration of other factors is incomplete and can be expected to have less than an optimal impact.

Approaches to Organization

In order to establish and maintain a regional perinatal care system, it is necessary to evaluate the existing state of maternal and child health in the region, identify unmet needs, institute a response, and evaluate results. On-site community and hospital surveys of personnel and facilities have been shown to be an effective tool in cataloging resources and examining consumer attitudes toward perceived needs and possible alterations in care practices. Responses to needs will vary but should be based on the following important considerations: (1) emphasis on local problem-solving by health care providers and consumers, (2) awareness of professional limitations by those charged with continuing education, (3) continued involvement of personal physicians and other providers in the care of their patients, and (4) outcome evaluation.

In many regions, a perinatal advisory group charged with the collaborative planning, implementation, and assessment of a comprehensive program has been effective. Regardless of the approach to development and institution of needed improvements in the system, continuity of commitment is essential. Education is the ultimate determinant of improved perinatal outcome. Effective communication, appropriate continuing education, and adequate funding require continual and consistent evaluation of data as the regional system of care evolves.

Risk Identification

Risk assessment and management, essential components of comprehensive perinatal care, begin when a patient enters the system (Table 1-1) and continue as long as the patient is receiving care. For maximum effectiveness, patients must enter the system as early as possible postconception. Most patients enter the system through their personal physician and their associations with the community hospital. This permits prospective selection of patients who might benefit from evaluation or care by another practitioner or institution.

Physicians in a region must work together to determine what constitutes additional risk, how to deal with that risk most effectively, and what the best alternatives are for present and future care in a region. This coordinated process facilitates acceptance of the resulting system of consultation, referral, and transfer.

Not all high-risk factors are discernible prior to labor or delivery. Therefore, all facilities that provide perinatal services should have the ability to detect unanticipated maternal, fetal, and neonatal complications and respond with timely, definitive care. For example, all sites in a perinatal system should have the capability to resuscitate and stabilize asphyxiated infants.

Problem Areas

The responsibilities of health professionals, especially obstetricians and pediatricians, in the care of the mother, fetus, and neonate have increasingly been viewed as complementary. Without mutual understanding, however, individual professional egos can hinder cooperative ventures such as regionalization. Hospitals and other institutions, agencies, and organizations may have vested interests that can also impede progress in this direction.

The values and strengths of local individual treatment should prevail in systematic and regionalized care. It should be made clear to providers that every part of the system supports personal attention to the patient and that the original primary care physician-patient relationship continues when referral or consultative care is no longer necessary. Therefore, continuing communication must be maintained. It should be made clear to consumers that the transfer of their trust to another provider is justified and that potential benefits outweigh whatever temporary family and community dislocation is necessary. Impersonal care can exist at any level but is justified at none.

Political divisions and geophysical boundaries often are barriers to regionalized perinatal health care. Similarly, the scattering of maternal and child health programs through multiple departments and agencies at the state and national levels of government has made refinement of developed systems more difficult in some circumstances. Planning and funding for education activities and transport, particularly maternal-fetal transport, have been inadequate in many regions. Funds for patient care should coincide with patients' needs without concern for county, state, or national boundaries.

COMPONENTS OF A REGIONAL PROGRAM

All regional organization models for perinatal care have certain identifiable activities that should be integrated into a plan with goals and objectives as discussed previously. Some regional programs may include activities other than those listed:

I. Patient Care
  A. Ambulatory services
    1. Maternal-fetal assessment and care
    2. Genetic diagnosis and counseling
    3. Laboratory evaluation
    4. Special procedures (e.g., amniocentesis, ultrasound)
    5. Neonatal follow-up
  B. Inpatient services
    1. Maternal-fetal services, including intensive care
    2. Neonatal services, including intensive care and surgery
    3. Radiologic services
    4. Ultrasound
  C. Consultation and referral
  D. Transportation
    1. Maternal-fetal transport
    2. Neonatal transport
    3. Return
II. Education
  A. Preventive and public health
  B. Patient awareness and preparation
  C. Professional
    1. Undergraduate/graduate studies
    2. Postgraduate and continuing education
  D. Institutions
    1. Hospitals
    2. Public service agencies
  E. Government
III. Evaluation and Research
  A. Outcome, including follow-up
  B. Biomedical results
  C. Systems

IV. Administration
   A. Data collection
   B. Hospital surveys
   C. Consultation
   D. Systems management

The primary component of any systematic approach to quality health care is personnel. Because perinatal care is multidisciplinary, involving medical, nursing, paramedical, and nonmedical personnel, leadership and communication are extremely important. A physician director or codirector must have interest, training, and experience in perinatal medicine, as well as in administration. Most of the following personnel should also be available in each region.

The obstetrician or family physician, sometimes working with a certified nurse-midwife who practices as a member of a team, is responsible for prenatal care, including risk assessment. When high-risk patients are encountered, appropriate consultation or referral may be necessary. Pediatricians and subspecialists in neonatology should take part in decision-making processes that have an impact on the fetus and newborn. Labor and delivery should be attended by personnel appropriate to the level of need. (For more information regarding attendance at cesarean births or high-risk deliveries, see Intrapartum Care, Chapter 4.) Postpartum care of the family is also a cooperative effort.

The role of nurses in perinatal medicine has been expanding. Outpatient and hospital nurses now play vital professional roles at all levels of care, and these roles should be identified and structured within a team effort in risk assessment and care. Certified nurse-midwives, obstetric/gynecologic nurse-practitioners, neonatal or perinatal nurse-clinicians or specialists, and pediatric nurse-practitioners make important contributions to the development of regional networks, the management of normal and unanticipated perinatal events, and follow-up. Each regional program should consider employing a perinatal nurse coordinator to assist with educational, service, and administrative endeavors.

Socioeconomic factors are significant determinants of pregnancy outcome, and social workers should be members of perinatal teams. Perinatal services with a great many high-risk patients require full-time social workers with special skills in perinatal problem-solving.

Health care administrators with special expertise in perinatal care should be encouraged to participate in regional programs. Such individuals may represent hospital, government, or private agencies.

Institutions associated with perinatal systems include hospitals, academic centers, and private and government agencies. Community hospitals should function with academic medical centers and specialty units (e.g., children's hospitals) as integral components of the system. Faculties at academic centers should play a leadership role in implementing standards for patient care and professional education. State and local agencies or foundations should not be limited to a supportive role, but rather should participate in the system.

Transport systems are necessary for each regional system. They require cooperation between institutions, which is best structured by affiliation and transport agreements. Specific details of transport systems differ from region to region, but adjoining regions might agree to share services. Transport services should be available to all perinatal patients, regardless of point of origin, and should include both maternal-fetal and neonatal services, as well as return services. Chapter 8 is devoted to this vital subject.

Funding guarantees are important to most effective regional systems. Although direct and third party payers can and should be expected to bear the cost of care and transport, these sources seldom provide adequate funding for other activities, such as education, research, and administration. Hospitals and academic institutions cannot be expected to subsidize these activities, however. Government agencies may help identify and solve funding problems. Progressive regional programs must anticipate the need for financial support and plan accordingly.

Education and training are essential components of regional programs. Academic centers working with community hospitals often provide this service, or it may be provided by integrated perinatal committees or associations of professional groups. Experience has shown that it is best to include personnel from as many parts of the system as possible, including levels I, II, and III.

Research and outcome surveillance should be integral parts of a regional program. The earlier discussion of goals and objectives elaborates upon this activity. Academic centers, nonacademic but tertiary level care institutions, the state vital statistics office, and the Bureau of Maternal and Child Health may share this responsibility. Periodic statistical summaries are very helpful.

THE FUTURE

In the future, regionally accepted protocols for specific perinatal problems will result from improved knowledge, education, and communication. Standardization of care will reflect regional needs. The acceptance of risk assessment as a process by which problems can be identified prior to labor and delivery will be increased. Perinatal care will be increasingly multidisciplinary, with more involvement of nonphysician members of the team. Level II program development and implementation will continue. Specialist obstetricians and pediatricians will collaborate with subspecialist maternal-fetal and neonatology associates located at level III or at regional resource centers.

Specialty areas, such as genetic and infertility counseling, will become increasingly important in regional perinatal programs. As prepregnancy and follow-up concerns are recognized, perinatal programs will evolve toward more comprehensive maternal and child health care.

The perinatal data base will increase, making it easier to identify those specific resources, including primary and specialty medical care, that improve reproductive outcome. Aided by better application of computer technology, this data base should facilitate regional planning and program implementation, as well as public education. A more comprehensive perinatal data base will be helpful in efforts to create individual and media interest in regionalized care. Concerted efforts will be necessary to interpret mortality and morbidity data and relate such data to cost factors.

Perinatal medicine will be increasingly dynamic and progressive as technology advances and knowledge of pathophysiology and human reproductive behavior increases. Authorities agree that present knowledge does not support extensive or rapid change in perinatal practice; further research is required. If investigation and evaluation yield reliable information on beneficial changes in birthing practice, such changes will need to be applied by physicians and institutions. The perinatal system described is flexible enough to incorporate appropriate changes.

RESOURCES AND RECOMMENDED READING

Aubry RH, Pennington JC: Identification and evaluation of high-risk pregnancy: The perinatal concept. Clin Obstet Gynecol 16:3–27, 1973

Bowes WA Jr: A review of perinatal mortality in Colorado, 1971 to 1978, and its relationship to the regionalization of perinatal services. Am J Obstet Gynecol 141(8):1045–1052, 1981

Butterfield LJ: Newborn country USA. Clin Perinatol 3(2):281–296, 1976

Cohen RS, Stevenson DK, Malachowski N, et al: Favorable results of neonatal intensive care for very low-birth-weight infants. Pediatrics 69(5):621–625, 1982

American Academy of Pediatrics, Committee on Fetus and Newborn: Level II neonatal units. Pediatrics 66(5): 810–811, 1980

American Academy of Pediatrics, Committee on Fetus and Newborn: Level II neonatal units. Pediatrics 66(5): 810–811, 1980

Harris TR, Isaman J, Giles HR: Improved neonatal survival through maternal transport. Obstet Gynecol 52(3):294–300, 1978

Harvey K, Bowes WA Jr: Maternal-fetal transport: Reflections on experience at University of Colorado. Perinatol-Neonatol 5(6):53–59, 1981

Hein HA: Evaluation of rural perinatal care system. Pediatrics 66(4): 540–546, 1980

Hein HA: The quality of perinatal care in small rural hospitals. JAMA 240(19):2070–2072, 1978

Hobel CJ: Risk assessment in perinatal medicine. Clin Obstet Gynecol 21:287–295, 1978

Hobel CJ, Hyvarinen MA, Okada DM, et al: Prenatal and intrapartum high-risk screening: I. Prediction of the high-risk neonate. Am J Obstet Gynecol 117:1–9, 1973

Hobel CJ, Youkeles L, Forsythe A: Prenatal and intrapartum high-risk screening: II. Risk factors reassessed. Am J Obstet Gynecol 135:1051–1056, 1979

Koops BL, Morgan LJ, Battaglia, FC: Neonatal mortality risk in relation to birth-weight and gestational age: update. J Pediatr 101(6):969–977, 1982

Ledger WJ: Identification of the high-risk mother and fetus—does it work? Clin Perinatol 7(1):125–134, 1980

McCarthy BJ, et al: Identifying neonatal risk factors and predicting neonatal deaths in Georgia. Am J Obstet Gynecol 142(5):557–562, 1982

National Foundation–March of Dimes, Committee on Perinatal Health: Toward Improving the Outcome of Pregnancy: Recommendations for the regional development of maternal and perinatal health services. White Plains, NY, National Foundation–March of Dimes, 1977

Paneth N, Kiely, JL, Wallenstein S, et al: Newborn intensive care and neonatal mortality in low-birth-weight infants: A population study. N Engl J Med 307:149–155, 1982 ·

Philip AGS, Little GA, Polivy DR, et al: Neonatal mortality risk for the eighties: The importance of birth-weight/gestational age groups. Pediatrics 68:122–130, 1981

Risk Approach for Maternal and Child Health Care: WHO Offset Publication No. 39. World Health Organization, Geneva, 1978

Ryan GM Jr, Fielden JG: The closure of maternity services in Massachusetts. Obstet Gynecol 52(3):369–370, 1978

Ryan GM Jr, Fielden JG: The impact of regionalization programs on patterns of perinatal care. Obstet Gynecol 53(2):187–189, 1979

Ryan GM Jr, Fielden JG, Pearse, WH: Regional planning–effects on the obstetrician-gynecologist. Obstet Gynecol 59(2):202–205, 1982

Sinclair JC, Lorrance GW, Boyle M, et al: Evaluating neonatal intensive care. Lancet 2:1052, 1981

Sinclair JC, Torrance GW, Boyle MH, et al: Evaluation of neonatal-intensive-care programs. N Engl J Med 305:489–494, 1981

Williams RL, Chen PM: Identifying the sources of the recent decline in perinatal mortality rates in California. N Engl J Med 306:207–214, 1982

2

Physical Facilities for Perinatal Care

Physical facilities for perinatal care in hospitals should be conducive to care that meets the normal physiologic and psychosocial needs of mothers and neonates. Special facilities should be available when deviations from normal require uninterrupted physiologic, biochemical, and clinical observation throughout the perinatal period. Contiguous location of areas for labor, delivery, and newborn care not only facilitates the necessary integration of obstetric, anesthetic, nursing, and pediatric efforts, but also ensures that patients who are moved from one of these areas to another undergo minimal contact with other patients and personnel.

The recommendations in this chapter are intended as general guidelines; they should be flexible enough to meet local needs. Physical arrangements for perinatal care should conform in principle to these guidelines but need not adhere to them in each detail. It is recognized that individual problems of physical facilities for perinatal care may impede conformity with the recommendations suggested and that not all hospitals will have all functional units described in this chapter. Furthermore, depending on patient volume and patient care resources available, functional units need not always be separate rooms. Provisions for individual units should be consistent with the regionalized perinatal care system discussed in detail in Chapter 1.

FUNCTIONAL UNITS

Obstetrics

The inpatient obstetric service should provide a safe and comfortable environment for women to deliver and care for their newborns. The patient's personal needs and those of her newborn and family should be considered when the service units are planned. The service should be consolidated in a designated area that, ideally, is physically separate from the remainder of the hospital, e.g., on a single floor or in an entire wing.

Functional obstetric (maternal) units may include the following facilities:

1. Admission/observation
2. Family waiting
3. Labor
4. Delivery/cesarean birth
5. Intensive care
6. Recovery
7. Birthing (combined labor/delivery/recovery)
8. Antepartum and postpartum beds
9. Sibling visitation

Hospitals providing level I services will not need an intensive care unit. Many of the other functional areas in these hospitals can be combined in a single room. The admission/examination area may serve as a labor room or recovery room, for example. Larger rooms may serve for labor/delivery/recovery, i.e., birthing rooms; other delivery rooms may be used for cesarean birth, and a family waiting room may be used for sibling visitation.

Facilities that provide level II care should contain all the functional units present in facilities that provide level I care, although more separate rooms may be justified by a larger volume of deliveries. All level III facilities provide intensive care, as do most level II facilities.

Labor and Delivery

ADMISSION/OBSERVATION. There should be a separate area designated in the admitting area for patient examination and short-term observation for patients who are not yet in active labor and for those who must be observed to determine whether labor has actually begun. A comfortable waiting area for the family should be adjacent to the labor and delivery suite.

LABOR. The number of beds required for labor is determined by the number of patients who have delivered in the past year. The number of beds should be adequate to handle the maximum patient load. As a general rule, one bed for labor can accommodate approximately 250 deliveries per year. More will be needed if they are used for antepartum observation and postpartum recovery as well as for women in active labor.

Single rooms with a window are recommended; the desirable size is 140 sq ft. If multiple occupancy is necessary, partitions or curtains are essential to ensure privacy. It is preferable that each bed in multibed rooms be allotted 100 sq ft of floor space. The door should be wide enough for a bed to pass through it. Local regulations concerning size and use of rooms vary; however, labor rooms may be planned so that they can be used for intensive care of high-risk patients in hospitals where there is no designated high-risk unit.

Following is a list of essential facilities for each labor room:

1. A labor or birthing bed with large wheels, adjustable side rails, removable head and foot boards, and a footstool
2. One or more comfortable chairs
3. Adjustable lighting that is pleasant for the patient and adequate for examinations
4. An emergency signal and an intercommunication system
5. Adequate ventilation and temperature control
6. Auxiliary electric system
7. A sphygmomanometer, stethoscope, and fetoscope
8. Mechanical infusion equipment
9. Capability for use of electronic fetal monitoring equipment
10. Oxygen and suction outlets
11. Hand-washing facilities in or immediately adjacent to each labor room
12. Conveniently located toilet facilities, which may be shared by two patients in different labor rooms
13. A writing surface for charting
14. Storage facilities for bedpans and supplies

The following additional facilities are needed in the labor room area:

1. A safe storage area for the patient's clothing and personal belongings
2. An instrument cleanup area
3. A preparation area and clean storage area
4. Area and equipment for bedpan cleansing
5. A secure area for medication storage
6. A nurses' station
7. Physician and nurse charting area

8. Conference room (desirable)

9. Staff lounge

Additional supplies and equipment in the labor and delivery room area may include the following items:

1. Stretcher with side rails
2. X-ray view boxes
3. Routine medications
4. Needles
5. Syringes
6. Solutions and equipment for administering fluids
7. Equipment for obtaining blood specimens
8. Ultrasound equipment

A central area in which medications can be prepared for patients in both the labor and delivery rooms is necessary. All drugs necessary to deal with emergencies that may arise during labor should be stocked in the labor and delivery area. Cardiopulmonary resuscitation carts should be available to carry the following items:

1. Needles
2. Syringes
3. Emergency drugs
4. Laryngoscope
5. Airways
6. Equipment for delivering positive pressure oxygen
7. Maternal cardiac monitor
8. Defibrillator

DELIVERY/CESAREAN BIRTH. In order to afford easy access, the delivery rooms should be contiguous to the labor rooms; however, they should be away from the entrance to the labor and delivery suite, and there should be no traffic through them. The number of delivery/cesarean birth rooms required depends on the average number of deliveries per day. Every delivery unit should have no less than two delivery rooms. It is widely accepted that four delivery rooms, one of which should be equipped for cesarean delivery, should be adequate for 3000 annual deliveries. An obstetric service of 1000–2000 deliveries would require two to three delivery rooms. Small obstetric services may consider equipping a labor room for alternate use as a delivery room.

It is desirable that cesarean deliveries be performed in the delivery unit and that postpartum sterilization capabilities be available. At least one delivery room should be equipped with an operating table and instruments necessary for emergency surgical obstetric intervention.

A delivery/cesarean birth room is similar to an operating room in design; a room with 350–400 sq ft open floor space with a ceiling height of 9 ft is adequate for normal or cesarean delivery. Each room should be equipped with the safeguards necessary for the administration of all forms of anesthesia. It should be adequately lighted and air-conditioned, and there should be an auxiliary electrical system. Room temperature should be controlled to prevent chilling of mother and neonate.

Each delivery/cesarean room should be maintained as a separate unit with equipment and supplies necessary for normal delivery and for the management of complications.

The following equipment and supplies are necessary:

1. A delivery table that allows variation in position for delivery
2. Instrument table and solution basin stand
3. Adequate lighting for vaginal or cesarean delivery
4. Instruments and equipment for vaginal delivery, repair of lacerations, cesarean delivery, and for the management of obstetric emergencies
5. Solutions and equipment for administering intravenous fluids
6. Equipment for inhalation and regional anesthesia, including equipment for emergency resuscitation
7. Heated, temperature-controlled neonatal examination and resuscitation unit
8. Equipment for examination, immediate care, and identification of the neonate
9. Individual oxygen, air, and suction outlets for mother and neonate
10. An emergency call system
11. Mirrors for patients to observe the birth
12. Wall clock with second hand

In addition, trays containing drugs and equipment necessary for emergency treatment of both mother and neonate should be kept in the delivery room area. Equipment necessary for the treatment of cardiac arrest should also be easily accessible.

The following auxiliary facilities should be available:

1. Scrub-up facilities. Scrub sinks, with hot and cold water and with

arm, knee, or foot controls should be placed so that, while scrubbing, the physician can observe the patient.

2. A workroom in which instruments are washed, and a separate room for preparing and sterilizing instruments. These rooms should be located near the delivery/cesarean birth room unless these services are provided by a central supply facility.

3. A room for storing supplies and equipment used in the labor and delivery area.

4. Laboratory facilities with a 24-hour capacity to provide blood group, Rh type and cross-matching, and basic emergency laboratory evaluations. Either type-compatible Rh specific or type O, Rh-negative blood should be available at the facility at all times. Other laboratory procedures, such as serologic testing and rubella titers, should be available.

INTENSIVE CARE. Patients who have significant medical or obstetric complications should be cared for in a room especially equipped with cardiopulmonary resuscitation equipment and other monitoring equipment necessary to allow observation and special care. This room may be located in the labor and delivery area and should meet the physical requirements of any other intensive care room in the hospital.

RECOVERY. On larger services, there should be a specific recovery room for postpartum patients with a separate area for high-risk patients. Generally, the number of recovery beds should be equal to one-half the number of labor beds. When a separate area is not possible, recently delivered patients should be observed by designated nursing personnel in a labor or delivery room.

The equipment needed is similar to that in any surgical recovery room and includes equipment for monitoring vital signs, suction, and administration of oxygen and intravenous fluids. Cardiopulmonary resuscitation equipment should be readily available.

BIRTHING (LABOR/DELIVERY/RECOVERY). To accommodate those women who want to deliver their babies in a more home-like setting but also want to have ready access to modern obstetric facilities, a birthing room may be used. The room should be a combined labor/delivery/recovery room where family members or other supporting persons may remain with a woman as much as possible throughout the childbirth process. It should be located in or close to the intrapartum area.

Furnishings should be bright, attractive, and comfortable with a modern labor and delivery bed that can be raised, lowered, and adjusted to a semi-sitting position and can be moved to the delivery/cesarean birth room if the need arises. A comfortable lounge chair is desirable. The room should contain the same equipment and supplies as other labor rooms, including equipment for electronic fetal monitoring, administering anesthesia, maintaining the neonate's temperature or warming the neonate, and administering oxygen. Preferably equipment should be concealed behind wall cabinets or drapes, but it must be readily available when needed.

Postpartum Unit

The number of beds required in a postpartum unit is determined by multiplying the number of annual deliveries by the average length of stay, and dividing by 365 days times the estimated occupancy rate:

$$\frac{\text{Annual deliveries} \times \text{Average stay}}{365 \times \text{Occupancy rate}} = \text{Number of postpartum beds}$$

This calculation does not provide for antepartum patients using these beds. A projected 85% occupancy rate minimizes overload beyond total bed capacity of the institution. The unit should be flexible enough to permit comfortable accommodation of the peak census and use of beds for alternate functions during low census. Ideally, not more than two patients should share one room.

Each patient unit should accommodate the patient, her newborn, and visitors without crowding. The minimum floor area for each bed should be approximately 100 sq ft in multibed rooms. There should be a minimum of 3 ft 8 in. between beds. Partitions or curtains are essential in multibed rooms to ensure privacy. Each unit should provide comfort, privacy, and protection against infection and other complications, as well as an atmosphere conducive to rest.

Each patient unit should include the following items:

1. Bed with adjustable side rails
2. Adequate lighting
3. Bedside stand
4. Space for clothes and personal belongings
5. Signal or intercommunication device
6. Bathing, toilet, and hand-washing facilities in or close to the patient's room and equipped with an emergency call signal.

If possible, each room should have its own toilet and washing facility; at least one toilet must be provided for every four patients or two rooms. It should be located close to the patients' rooms, and patients should be able to reach it without entering a general corridor.

When rooming-in is permitted, each room should have hand-washing facilities, a mobile bassinet unit, and supplies necessary for the care of the newborn.

A sibling visitation room adjacent to the postpartum area is desirable to accommodate older children's visits with mothers confined to the antepartum and postpartum area, as allowed by state and local regulations.

Supporting Service Areas

In addition to those already mentioned, each postpartum unit should include the following facilities:

1. A nurses' station
2. Physician and nurse charting area
3. Washroom for staff use
4. An examining and treatment room
5. A kitchen or pantry from which food may be served to the patients (optional)
6. Clean-up area
7. Area for medication preparation
8. Patient education area
9. Adequate clean storage and preparation area
10. Conference room
11. Lounge for patients and visitors
12. Sitz bath facilities

The following equipment should be available:

1. Sphygmomanometers and stethoscopes
2. Intravenous solution and infusion supplies
3. Catheter equipment and supplies
4. Stretcher with side rails
5. Emergency drugs
6. Cardiopulmonary resuscitation cart

Locker, rest room, and sleeping facilities for personnel should be located near the entrance to the labor and delivery area. Doors from these areas should open into a corridor outside the labor and delivery suite as well as directly into it. The facilities should be comfortable, quiet, and, when necessary, air-conditioned. Individual lockers, toilets, and showers should be available. Comfortable chairs and beds should be provided.

In addition to lockers, showers, and toilets, separate sleeping rooms and a lounge are necessary for physicians. The sleeping room should contain enough comfortable beds to accommodate those physicians who must be in the hospital because they have patients in labor. The lounge should be furnished with comfortable chairs and should be provided with dictating equipment.

Pediatrics

Pediatric functional units include the following areas:

1. Resuscitation
2. Admission/observation
3. Normal newborn care
4. Continuing care
5. Intermediate care
6. Intensive care
7. Parent-neonate visitation

Level I facilities should provide areas for resuscitation, admission/observation, normal newborn care, and parent-neonate visitation. Some level I facilities may provide continuing care for neonates with relatively uncomplicated problems that do not require sophisticated laboratory, radiographic, or pediatric consultative services. Hospitals with level II services should provide the same areas, plus areas designated for continuing care and intermediate care. Level III facilities should have intensive care areas in addition to all other pediatric areas.

In Table 2-1, the bed requirements, space needs, and nurse/patient ratios for service areas provided within the regionalized system of neonatal care are summarized. The number of beds may be distributed among several hospitals in a region. For example, a region with 25,000 deliveries may require 25 beds for intensive care, 75–100 beds for intermediate neonatal care, and 50 beds for continuing neonatal care. These beds can be distributed among all the appropriately qualified facilities in the region.

In the design of neonatal facilities, it may occasionally be undesirable to establish physically separated patient care areas, i.e., intensive, intermediate, and continuing care areas. For economy of personnel, as well as for primary care nursing, consideration should be given

Table 2–1. Bed Requirements, Space Needs, and Nurse/Patient Ratios for Service Areas in Neonatal Care

Service or facility provided	Levels of care I	Levels of care II	Levels of care III	Beds needed per 1000 deliveries*	Space needs (sq ft/bed)	Nurse/patient ratio
Delivery/resuscitation	x	x	x	1	120	1:1
Admission/observation	x	x	x	2	40	1:4
Normal newborn	x	x	x	10–12†	20	1:6–8
Postpartum new family unit	x	x	x	10–12†	100	1:3 (mother/newborn pairs)
Intermediate care		x	x	3–4	50	1:3–4
Continuing/convalescent care	††	x	x	2	30	1:4
Intensive care		††	x	1	80–100	1:1–2

*These figures are based on a prematurity rate of 80/1000 births. If adjustment is required, the actual prematurity rate per 1000 can be divided by 80 and the result multiplied by the number in the table. For example, if the prematurity rate per 1000 is 120, the number of intermediate care beds needed is 6: (120 ÷ 80) × 4 = 6.

†Bed needs can be divided between newborn nursery and postpartum new family unit, depending on requests for type of service.

††Optionally, these functional units may be provided if there is a demand for such service and the hospital is able to provide laboratory, radiologic, and other pediatric consultative services as well as physical facilities.

to a mix of patients in a single area so that nurses can care for neonates who are extremely ill as well as for those who are less severely ill. Local circumstances should be considered in the design and management of patient care areas.

Patient Care Areas

RESUSCITATION. It is in the resuscitation area that neonates are resuscitated and stabilized immediately after birth. Depending on their condition, neonates go from this area to the admission/observation area, the intermediate care area, or the intensive care area in the same hospital, or they are transferred to an intermediate care or intensive care area in a hospital providing level II or level III care.

The resuscitation area should be lighted so the illumination is at least 100 foot-candles at the neonate's body surface. It should contain the following items:

1. Overhead source of radiant heat
2. Heating pad overlying a thin mattress on which the neonate is placed
3. Large wall clock with a clearly visible second hand
4. Flat working surface for charting
5. Table or flat surface for trays and equipment that may be needed
6. Equipment for endotracheal intubation, administration of compressed oxygen and air, umbilical vessel catheterization, and transfusion procedures

Although the resuscitation area may be within the delivery/cesarean birth room, a designated separate room next to or opening into the delivery/cesarean birth room is desirable. If resuscitation is done within a delivery/cesarean birth room, the area should be large enough to ensure that resuscitation of the neonate does not interfere with maternal care. Following stabilization of the neonate, if the mother wishes to hold her newborn, a radiant heater or prewarmed blankets should be available to keep the neonate warm.

The amount of space required for a resuscitation room is approximately 120 sq ft, or a minimum of 40 sq ft within a delivery/cesarean birth room. The area should have one suction outlet, one oxygen outlet, one compressed air outlet, and at least six electrical outlets with a capacity of 15 amp. In addition, a separate resuscitation room should have an electrical outlet to accommodate a portable x-ray machine, as needed. Electrical outlets should conform to the regulations for areas in which anesthetic agents are administered.

A detailed list of equipment and supplies required for resuscitation is in Appendix B. The equipment and required drugs should be checked by a designated individual following delivery and at least once each nursing shift.

ADMISSION/OBSERVATION (TRANSITIONAL CARE STABILIZATION). The admission/observation area is for careful evaluation of the neonate's condition during the first 4–24 hours after birth, i.e., during the period of physiologic adjustment to extrauterine life. This evaluation may take place within one or more functional areas, e.g., the mother's recovery room, the birthing room, the newborn nursery, or a separate admission/observation area. In some hospitals, newborn nurseries are primary areas for transitional care, both for neonates born within the hospital and those born outside the hospital. No separate isolation facilities are required for neonates born at home or in transit to the hospital.

The admission/observation area should be near or adjacent to the delivery/cesarean birth room. If it is part of the maternal recovery area, which is preferable, physical separation of mother and newborn during this period can be avoided. In level I facilities, the admission/observation area may also function as a resuscitation area. In level II and III facilities, the admission/observation area may be located in the newborn or continuing care area if a separate room is not provided.

An estimated 40 sq ft is needed for each neonate in this area. The capacity required depends on the size of the delivery service and the duration of close observation. One patient station for each 300 annual births is needed if the length of stay in the area is 24 hours. Fewer stations are needed if the stay is of shorter duration, but there should be a minimum of two stations in this area. The admission/observation area should be well lighted, have a large wall clock, and be equipped to provide emergency resuscitation similar to that provided in the resuscitation area. Outlets should also be similar to those in the resuscitation area.

The physicians' and nurses' assessment of neonates determines the level of care that follows. Most neonates go from the admission/observation area to the newborn nursery area or the postpartum area for rooming-in. Some neonates require transfer to an intermediate or intensive care area.

NEWBORN NURSERY. Routine nursery care of apparently normal full-term or preterm neonates who weigh more than 2000 g at birth and have demonstrated successful adaptation to extrauterine life is provided in the newborn care area. This area should be close to the postpartum rooms. In a multifloor maternity unit, there should be a newborn care area on each floor.

The number of bassinets should exceed the obstetric beds by 25% to accommodate multiple births, extended neonatal hospitalization, and a fluctuating patient load. Required capacity can also be estimated based on the mean duration of stay and annual number of liveborn, normal, full-term, and preterm neonates. For example, if these neonates are in the hospital an average of 3 days, each bassinet has a capacity of 120 neonates (365 ÷ 3 = 120). If the average number of normal live births is 2000, an average of 17 bassinets (2000 ÷ 120 = 17) are always in use. Adding 25% additional bassinets for fluctuations in patient census indicates that 20 or 21 bassinets are required for this unit.

Because the care in this area is provided by relatively few persons and there is no need for bulky equipment, 20 sq ft for each neonate should be adequate. There must be at least 2 ft between bassinets in all directions, measured from the edge of one bassinet to the edge of the adjacent one. Institutions considering remodeling or new facilities may wish to consider 30 sq ft for each neonate with 3 ft between bassinets, depending on local considerations, such as the presence of nursing and medical students in the nursery. The newborn care area may be in one room in a small hospital or in one or more rooms in larger hospitals. Because one nursing staff member is required for each 6–8 neonates, individual rooms should have accommodations for 6–8, 12–16, or 18–24 neonates.

The area must be well lighted, have a large wall clock, and be equipped for emergency resuscitation. One pair of wall-mounted electrical outlets is recommended for each two neonatal stations, and one oxygen outlet, one compressed air outlet, and one suction outlet are recommended for each five or six neonatal stations.

Cabinets and counters within the newborn care area should be available for storage of routinely used supplies, such as diapers, formula, linens, and gauze. The following supplies that may be conveniently stored within or near the bassinet:

1. Thermometer with lubricant
2. Towelettes
3. Diapers
4. Shirts

5. Blankets
6. Linen
7. Soap
8. Lotion
9. Cottonballs
10. Alcohol
11. Applicators
12. Tape measure

CONTINUING CARE. Low-birth-weight neonates who are not sick but require frequent feeding, and neonates who no longer require intermediate care but still require more hours of nursing than normal neonates should be taken to the continuing care area. This area should be close to the intensive and intermediate care areas.

Because the care of neonates in this area requires some bulky equipment (e.g., rocking chairs and stools), as well as more personnel than are needed in the newborn nursery, more space is needed. There should be 30 sq ft for each patient station with approximately 3 ft between bassinets or incubators. When making plans for remodeling or acquiring new facilities, institutions may wish to consider providing 40 sq ft for each neonate with 4 ft between bassinets, depending on such factors as the number of parents, students, and other personnel expected to be in the unit.

The number of beds for continuing care needed in a region is determined by the number of neonates who require intensive or intermediate care, plus the number of neonates who do not require intensive or intermediate care but need increased nursing time. For example, the level II and III facilities in a region with a low-birth-weight delivery rate of 80/1000 births needs about two beds for continuing care per 1000 births (Table 2–1). This figure can be modified according to the neonatal risk in a particular region.

As in the resuscitation and admission/observation areas, equipment for emergency resuscitation is required in this area. It may be most conveniently kept within an emergency cart or cabinet, but it should be readily available when necessary. There should be four electrical outlets, one oxygen outlet, one compressed air outlet, and one suction outlet for each neonatal station. In addition, equipment and supplies necessary for the newborn area should be available in the continuing care area. Provisions should be made for the comfort of parents or personnel who feed neonates in both incubators and bassinets.

INTERMEDIATE CARE. Sick neonates who do not require intensive care but require 6–12 nursing hours each day should be taken to the intermediate care area. The following recommendations represent the minimum facilities required to provide intermediate care; they are not intended for hospitals that provide assisted ventilation for prolonged periods of time in this area.

The intermediate care area should be close to the delivery/cesarean birth room and the intensive care area, and it should be away from general hospital traffic. It should have radiant heaters or incubators for maintaining body temperature, as well as infusion pumps, cardiopulmonary monitors, and equipment needed for the level of ventilatory assistance provided.

The number of beds for intermediate care for a region is determined by the number of neonates who have required intensive care, plus the number of neonates who need an intermediate level of care from the outset. Level II and III hospitals in a region with a low-birthweight delivery rate of 80/1000 births need about three beds for intermediate care per 1000 births. This number of beds should be corrected by a factor reflecting the level of risk for neonates born in the particular region (Table 2–1).

An estimated 50 sq ft are needed for every patient station. Additional space, e.g., for desks, counters, cabinets, corridors, and treatment rooms should be added to the space needed for patients. There should be at least 4 ft between incubators, bassinets, or radiant heaters in intermediate care areas. Aisles should be 5 ft wide.

Neonates receiving intermediate care may be housed in a single large room or in two or more rooms. In the latter case, each room should accommodate some multiple of three infant stations, because one nursing staff member is generally required for every three or four intermediate care patients. Large rooms allow greater flexibility in the use of equipment and assignment of personnel.

Eight electrical outlets, two oxygen outlets, two compressed air outlets, and two suction outlets should be provided for each patient station. In addition, the area should be provided with a special outlet to power the neonatal unit's portable x-ray machine.

All equipment and supplies for resuscitation should be immediately available and present within the intermediate care unit. These may be conveniently placed in an emergency cart (Appendix B).

INTENSIVE CARE. Constant nursing and continuous cardiopulmonary and other support for severely ill infants should be provided in the intensive care area. Because emergency care is provided in this area, laboratory and radiologic facilities must be readily available 24 hours/ day. The intensive care area preferably should be near the delivery/ cesarean birth room and should be within easy access from the ambulance entrance. It should be away from routine hospital traffic. Intensive care may be administered in a single area, or it can be provided in two or more separate rooms, each with a capacity of four or more infants.

The number of beds for intensive care for a region with a low-birth-weight delivery rate of 80/1000 live births is one bed per 1000 births. This figure should be adjusted for each region's low-birth-weight delivery rate (Table 2–1). Not only the number of nursing, medical, and surgical personnel, but also the amount and complexity of equipment required, is considerably greater in intensive care areas than in other perinatal areas. Therefore, there should be at least 6 ft between incubators, and aisles should be 8 ft wide. The area should have 80–100 sq ft for each neonate, plus space for such things as desks, cabinets, and corridors. In addition, the educational responsibilities of a Level III facility require that the design of its intensive care area include space for instructional activities and office space for data files on the region's perinatal activities.

Each patient station needs 12–16 electrical outlets, 2–4 oxygen outlets, 2–4 compressed air outlets, and 2–3 suction outlets. All electrical outlets for each patient station should be on both regular and auxiliary power. In addition, the area should be provided with a special outlet to power the neonatal unit's portable x-ray machine.

Equipment and supplies in the intensive care area should include all that is necessary for the resuscitation and intermediate care areas. Supplies should be kept close to the patient station so that nurses are not away from the neonate unnecessarily and nursing time and skills are used efficiently. A central modular supply system can enhance efficiency. In addition, equipment for long-term ventilatory support should be provided. Respirators should be equipped with nebulizers or humidifiers with heaters. Continuous on-line monitoring of oxygen concentrations, body temperature, and blood pressure should be available.

In some situations, a treatment room for the performance of minor surgical procedures may be desirable. Equipment, facilities, and supplies for this area, as well as procedures, must conform or be comparable to those required for similar procedures in the surgical department of the hospital.

Visitation

Mothers and fathers should have access to their newborns 24 hours/
day within all functional units and should be encouraged to participate
in the care of their newborns. Generally, parents can be with their
newborns in the mothers' rooms.

Special provisions may be necessary when neonates are in special
care units, i.e., continuing, intermediate, or intensive care. In these
situations, mothers are often discharged from the hospital before their
newborns and sometimes must travel long distances to be with them.
The needs of parents and their newborns under these circumstances
should be given careful consideration. Several systems have been
developed to meet these needs, e.g., parents' rooms with beds in the
hospital, adjacent facilities outside the hospital but provided by the
hospital, or motel facilities near the hospital. Each institution should
develop its own system to foster internal family relationships while a
neonate is receiving special care; this is an important aspect of neonatal
care that may help to prevent the complications of child care, child
abuse, and child neglect, which frequently involve neonates discharged
from special care units. A period of mother-newborn rooming-in prior
to discharge is also highly desirable.

Sibling visitation of the mother may be encouraged and should
take place in the mother's private room or a specially designed room.
The father or another adult should accompany the siblings and assume
responsibility for their care and conduct. Guidelines for sibling visitation should be developed by nursing, pediatric, obstetric, and infectious disease personnel.

Supporting Service Areas

UTILITY ROOMS. Both "clean" and "dirty" utility rooms are needed. A
clean utility area is for preparing formulas, medications, and supplies
frequently used in the care of neonates in all functional units. The use
of ready-mixed formulas, disposable supplies and equipment, and
unit-dose medications has lessened the need for clean utility rooms,
and this area may be replaced by storage areas and clean working
surfaces within each functional unit in intermediate and intensive care
areas.

A dirty utility area is for storing soiled and contaminated material
before its removal from the nursery area. This generally includes
equipment that is resterilized in a central service department. Contam-

inated equipment may be decontaminated in the dirty utility area and transported to the central service department in plastic bags or containers. These and other contaminated materials should be removed from the nursery on a regular basis. Contaminated linen should not be stored in the dirty utility area, but should be taken directly from the nursery in plastic or other nonporous containers to appropriate hospital facilities.

The dirty utility rooms should contain a counter and a sink with hot and cold running water that is turned on and off by knee or foot controls, soap and paper towel dispensers, a covered waste receptacle with foot control, and space for storage of contaminated equipment prior to its removal. A separate sink or hopper with hot and cold running water should be available for cleaning equipment prior to its return to the central service department for sterilization.

STORAGE AREAS. A system that provides three progressive levels of storage is desirable. The first storage area should be the central supply department of the hospital. The second storage area should be adjacent to or within the patient care areas. In this area, routinely used supplies, such as diapers, formula, linen, cover gowns, charts, and information booklets, may be stored. The quantity depends on the operation of the central supply department of the hospital. Generally, space is required only for the amount of each item used between supply deliveries, e.g., daily or three times weekly. The third area of storage is for frequently used items at the neonate's bedside, e.g., bassinet, warmer, or incubator.

Bedside cabinet storage should be approximately 8 cu ft for each patient unit in the newborn nursery, 16 cu ft for each patient unit in the intermediate care area, and 24 cu ft for each patient unit in the intensive care area. The newborn nursery requires approximately 3 cu ft/patient for secondary storage of items such as linen and formula. There should be approximately 8 cu ft of secondary storage space for each patient for syringes, needles, intravenous infusion sets, and sterile trays needed in such procedures as umbilical vessel catheterization, lumbar puncture, and thoracostomy in the resuscitation, admission/ observation, continuing care, intermediate care, and intensive care areas.

Large items of equipment, e.g., bassinets, warmers, radiant heaters, phototherapy units, and infusion pumps, should be stored in a clean storage area. Approximately 6 sq ft of floor space for each patient is required for equipment for the newborn area, 18 sq ft for the intermediate care area, and 30 sq ft for the intensive care area.

TREATMENT ROOMS. The need for a separate treatment room for the performance of procedures such as lumbar punctures, intravenous infusions, venipuncture, and minor surgical procedures has been largely eliminated with the development of resuscitation, admission/observation, intermediate care, and intensive care areas. Each patient station in these areas constitutes a treatment area in itself. However, if neonates in the newborn nursery, continuing care area, or the postpartum new family unit are to undergo certain procedures, e.g., circumcision, a separate treatment area may be required. The facilities, outlets, equipment, and supplies should be similar to those of the resuscitation area. The amount of space required depends on the number of procedures performed. Level I facilities may be served by a single treatment room with 120 sq ft, whereas level II and level III facilities should have an additional 40 sq ft/1000 live births.

SCRUB AREAS. At the entrance to each nursery, there should be a scrub area adequate to accommodate all personnel entering the area. It should be supplied with a sink large enough to prevent splashing. Foot- or knee-operated controls should be available. Sinks for hand-washing should not be built into counters used for other purposes. The scrub areas should also contain racks, hooks, or lockers for storing street clothing and personal items. There should also be cabinets for clean gowns, a receptacle for used gowns, and a large wall clock with a sweep second hand for timing hand-washing.

Scrub sinks with foot- or knee-operated controls should also be provided for at least each five or six patient stations in the newborn nursery, for every three patient stations in the intermediate care area, and for every two patient stations in the intensive care area. In addition, one scrub sink is needed in the resuscitation area, and one is needed for every three to four patient stations in the admission/observation and continuing care areas.

NEWBORN BATHING AREA. Newborns may be given a bath after their condition has stabilized and they have demonstrated an adequate adjustment to extrauterine life. This may be most conveniently performed in the admission/observation area or in the newborn nursery. In order to be large enough for newborn bathing, the sink should be 12 by 24 by 7 in. It should have knee- or foot-operated faucets and a flat surface for drying the neonate. Large, prewarmed absorbent towels and an overhead radiant heat source help to keep the infant warm. There should be no drafts or forced air vents in this area. Scales can be placed in this area for weighing the neonate after bathing. Daily baths may consist of sponge baths within the bassinet, as necessary.

NURSING AREAS. There are five functional units in the nursing areas:

1. Bedside. Space should be provided at the bedside not only for patient care, but also for education and charting activities. Charting should be considered an unclean procedure even when performed at the bedside, and when the activity has been completed, personnel should wash their hands before further contact with a neonate. Scrub sinks and a flat writing surface, e.g., a clipboard, are needed.

2. Charting area. A nurses' charting area or desk for tasks such as keeping more detailed records, completing requisitions, and handling specimens may be useful. Physicians may also perform charting and clerical activities in this area. Such areas should be located outside the functional units and should be considered unclean, i.e., personnel should wash their hands before further contact with infants.

3. Nursing offices. The nursing supervisor and head nurse should have offices close to the newborn care areas.

4. Dressing rooms. Close to the nursery entrance should be a nurses dressing room with lockers; storage for gowns, scrub dresses, and caps; hampers for disposal of used clothing; and toilet facilities.

5. Nurses' lounge. It is desirable to have a nurses' lounge adjacent to or connecting with the dressing room.

EDUCATION AREAS. A conference room suitable for education purposes is desirable in some level II and all level III facilities. This may be provided in the hospital adjacent to the maternity-newborn area.

CLERICAL AREAS. The control point for patient care activities is the clerical area; it should be located near the entrance to the nurseries so that the secretary can supervise traffic and limit unnecessary entry into the patient care areas. In addition, patients' charts and hospital forms may be stored in the clerical area. It should have telephones and intercommunications with the various neonatal care areas and the delivery suite.

General Considerations

ILLUMINATION. All newborn care areas should have 100 foot-candles of illumination. The system should provide light at variable intensities with deluxe cool white fluorescent bulbs.

WINDOWS. Solid, windowless walls provide the best temperature insulation for nurseries, but they may have a depressing effect on personnel. If there are windows, they should have untinted glass insulated with double panes. When possible, it may be preferable to utilize outside walls for nonpatient areas, e.g., storage, desks, or charting.

INTERIOR FINISH. Off-white or pale beige minimizes distortion of the staff's color perception in patient care areas. Brighter colors may be used elsewhere. Nursery windows should have off-white or pale beige window shades that match the interior color, are easy to clean, and are fireproof.

OXYGEN AND COMPRESSED AIR OUTLETS. Newborn care areas should have oxygen and compressed air piped from a central source at 50–60 psi. An alarm system should be included to warn of any critical reduction in line pressure. Reduction valves and mixers should produce 21%–100% concentrations of oxygen at atmospheric pressure for head hoods and 50–60 psi for mechanical ventilators.

ACOUSTIC CHARACTERISTICS. The ventilation system, monitors, incubators, suction pumps, mechanical ventilators, and staff produce considerable noise. The noise level should be monitored intermittently. Nursery construction and redesign should include acoustic absorption units or other means to keep sound intensity below 75 dB.

ELECTRICAL OUTLETS AND ELECTRICAL EQUIPMENT. All electrical outlets should have a common ground. Each patient station should have sufficient outlets to handle all pieces of equipment that might be needed by a patient at that station, and all outlets should be attached to the common ground. All electrical equipment should be checked for current leakage and grounding adequacy when first introduced into the nursery, at least once a month thereafter, and when combined with other equipment. The cord and cap of all electrical equipment should have a strain reliever. Plugs should be hospital grade.* Adaptors, extension cords, and junction boxes should not be used.

Although the amount of current leakage that is safe for neonates is not definitely known, leakage of more than 100μ amp from an array

---

*Hospital grade receptacles and plugs employ a conventional parallel blade with ground and are listed by the Underwriter's Laboratories, Inc. They are identified by the grounding symbol (=), the phrase *hospital grade*, and a green dot in the projecting face of the receptacle and on the face of the attachment plug.

of electrical devices should be avoided. No single item should have a current leakage of more than 10μ amp.

Labeling each outlet with the current capacity of the fuse or circuit breaker that serves it minimizes the chances of electrical failure from a circuit overload. Current capacity of each outlet should be at least twice the sum of the current rating of all the electrical equipment for which that outlet is used. Some electrical outlets in the nursery should be on the hospital's emergency circuit to maintain life support systems. The ground on these outlets must be the same as that for the other outlets.

Nursery personnel should be thoroughly and repeatedly instructed in the potential electrical hazards within the nursery.

SAFETY AND ENVIRONMENTAL CONTROL. The complexities in environmental control and monitoring require a hospital environmental engineer to ensure that all electrical, lighting, air composition, and temperature systems function properly and safely. Humidity should be between 40% and 60%; it should be controlled by the heating and air-conditioning system of the hospital.

RESOURCES AND RECOMMENDED READING

American College of Obstetricians and Gynecologists: Family-Centered Maternity/Newborn Care in Hospitals. Washington, DC, ACOG, 1978

American College of Obstetricians and Gynecologists: Standards for Obstetric/Gynecologic Services, 5 ed. Washington, DC, ACOG, 1982

National Foundation–March of Dimes, Committee on Perinatal Health: Toward Improving the Outcome of Pregnancy: Recommendations for the regional development of maternal and perinatal health services. White Plains, NY, National Foundation–March of Dimes, 1977

Ross Laboratories: Planning and Design for Perinatal and Pediatric Facilities. Columbus, OH, Ross Laboratories, 1977

Ross Planning Associates: Alternatives for Obstetric Design. Columbus, OH, Ross Laboratories, 1980

US Department of Health, Education, and Welfare; Public Health Service; Health Resources Administration; Bureau of Health Facilities Financing, Compliance, and Conversion: Minimum Requirements for Construction & Equipment for Hospital & Medical Facilities. DHEW Publication No: (HRA) 79-14500. Washington, DC, US Government Printing Office, 1979

3
Personnel for
Perinatal Services

Quality perinatal care requires adequate numbers of appropriately trained personnel. The staffing requirements of each hospital depend on its patient care commitments, the nature of the population it serves, and its education, evaluation, and research obligations. During the past decade, hospitals have been designated level I, II, or III on the basis of their personnel and capital investments in perinatal care services. Patient volume and availability of special services in the region have also been factors in these designations. More recent developments make it clear that programs within a single hospital may vary in complexity from level I to level III. Shared education, evaluation, research, and, in some cases, patient care facilities, are practical, economical alternatives. Although such arrangements do not change the basic staff needed by these hospitals to discharge their varied institutional responsibilities successfully, they do lead to more complex, multilayered arrangements within and between community care centers. It is with these thoughts in mind that the term *level of care* is employed in this chapter.

Hospitals committed to provide level I care should have an adequate staff for the following functions:

1. Surveillance and care of all patients admitted to the obstetric service
2. Care of postpartum conditions
3. Proper detection and supportive care of unexpected maternal-fetal problems that occur during labor and delivery
4. Performance of cesarean delivery
5. Effective resuscitation of all neonates born in their delivery facilities
6. Stabilization of unexpectedly small or sick neonates before transfer elsewhere

7. Evaluation of the condition of healthy neonates and continuing care for them until discharge

Hospitals committed to provide level II care should have not only staff to provide level I services, but also additional personnel to manage the problems of high-risk mothers and neonates, both from their own as well as outlying level I hospital obstetric services.

Hospitals providing level III services should have personnel to provide perinatal services for all mothers and neonates, regardless of risk assessment. In addition, sufficient personnel are necessary to carry out research needs adequately, as well as regional data-gathering analysis and evaluation.

Recommended nurse/patient ratios are shown in Table 3–1. If an institution has implemented a particular variable staffing system that has proved effective, it may be more appropriate to use it in order to meet specific institutional needs.

HOSPITALS PROVIDING LEVEL I SERVICES

Level I Medical Staff

One physician should be responsible for perinatal care. Where resources are available and separate responsibility for maternal-fetal and neonatal care is appropriate, the chiefs of the obstetric and pediatric services should be cochiefs of the program for perinatal care. This administrative approach requires close coordination and unified policy statements. Responsibilities include policy development, maintenance of standards of care, and consultation with staff at those hospitals providing levels II and III care in the region.

A qualified physician or a certified nurse-midwife should attend all deliveries. A physician who is responsible for the care of the neonate should also be available. A qualified anesthesiologist or nurse-anesthetist should be on call to administer appropriate anesthesia and maintain support of vital functions in any emergency.

Level I Nursing Staff

A registered nurse should be in charge of the nursing staff of the hospital's perinatal facilities. This nurse may also be responsible for directing nursing services and implementing policy in the labor and delivery, newborn care, and postpartum care areas.

A registered nurse who has training and competence in perinatal nursing; who can evaluate the condition of the mother, fetus, and

Table 3–1. *Recommended Nurse/Patient Ratios for Perinatal Services*

Staffing	Ratio	Care provided
Labor and delivery	1:2	Normal laboring patients
	1:1	Intensely ill patients with complications
	1:1	Patients in second stage
	1:2	Oxytocin induction or augmentation of labor
	1:1	Coverage of epidural anesthesia
	2:1	Cesarean deliveries (the circulating nurse should be a registered nurse)
	1:6–8	Patients in antepartum or postpartum areas
Nurseries		
Newborn nursery	1:6–8	Newborns needing only routine newborn ward care
	1:3	Mother-newborn units
Intermediate nursery	1:3–4	Intermediate care nursery
	1:4	Continuing convalescent care area
Newborn intensive care unit	1:1	Multisystem support, including ventilating support
	1:2	Critical care of unstable neonate

newborn infant; and who can assess the degree of risk to which they are subject during labor, delivery, and the neonatal period should always be present when a woman is in labor. Although there are significant fluxes in the number of women in labor at a given time in any hospital that has a low number of deliveries, the hospital should provide a qualified registered nurse to be in attendance at all times when there are patients in active labor in the unit. The recommended ratios are listed in Table 3–1.

A qualified person who can resuscitate and intubate neonates, if necessary, should be present at all deliveries.

Nursing personnel assigned to nursery areas in level I hospitals should be able to identify and alert physicians to pathophysiologic processes and oversee the immediate postpartum recovery period. They should also understand the environmental requirements of the newborn. In addition, they should be able to perform emergency procedures, such as resuscitation, and to provide intravenous or enteral nutrition. One member of the nursing staff is required on each shift for every four infants in the admission/observation area (6 hours care every 24 hours). If the same nurse is responsible for the resuscitation of neonates immediately after delivery as well as for the resuscitation of those in the nursery area, these areas should be adjacent. Additional personnel should be available for emergency situations.

Nursing personnel in the newborn care area should be under the direct supervision of a registered nurse. One member of the nursing staff is required on each shift for every six to eight neonates (3–4 hours care every 24 hours). This area should have housekeeping and other ancillary personnel to ensure that the nursing staff have time for their primary duties.

When several services are performed in one physical location, the supervising nurse on each shift may be directly responsible for labor and delivery, as well as resuscitation. In such a case, neonates in the special care and the normal care areas may be managed by other nursing staff under the supervising nurse's direction. In smaller hospitals, the same personnel may staff all of these areas.

Each hospital should have well-developed contingency plans with other hospitals within the system for those times in which the patient load is unusually heavy.

In addition to fulfilling the responsibilities associated with each functional area, the nursing staff of the perinatal service should be available to provide emotional support to parents, to make referrals for social services, and to instruct parents in neonate care practices.

HOSPITALS PROVIDING LEVEL II SERVICES

Level II Medical Staff

A board-certified obstetrician with special interest, experience, and, in some situations, special competence certification in maternal-fetal medicine should be chief of the obstetric service. A board-certified pediatrician with special interest, experience, and, in some situations, subspecialty certification in neonatal medicine should be chief of the newborn care service. These physicians should coordinate the hospital's perinatal services and, in conjunction with other medical, nursing, and hospital administration staff, should develop policies concerning staffing, routine procedures, equipment, and supplies.

In order to ensure the safe and effective administration of anesthesia, the director of anesthesia services should be board-certified and should have training and experience in obstetric anesthesia. A nurse-anesthetist or anesthesiologist with special competence and experience in obstetric anesthesia should be available 24 hours/day. Policies regarding the provision of obstetric anesthesia, including qualifications of personnel and availability for both routine and emergency deliveries, should be developed. The hospital staff should also include a radiologist and, optimally, a pathologist who are on call 24 hours/day. Specialized medical and surgical consultation should be readily available.

Level II Nursing Staff

A registered nurse with both education and experience in the management of normal as well as high-risk pregnancy, labor, and delivery should be solely responsible for the supervision of maternal-fetal nursing and implementation of policies in the level II labor, delivery, and postpartum areas. A registered nurse with education and experience in the treatment of sick neonates should be solely responsible for the supervision of neonatal nursing and implementation of policies in the neonatal care areas. These nurses should be assisted by an administrative coordinator responsible for staffing and training schedules, ordering of supplies, and maintenance of equipment. The administrative coordinator may be a registered nurse or another health professional with administrative experience.

Nursing staff in the labor, delivery, and recovery areas should be certified or experienced in identifying and responding to obstetric and medical complications of pregnancy, labor, and delivery. Staffing requirements for the resuscitation, admission/observation, and newborn care areas are the same as those for hospitals that provide level I care.

The nursing staff of the intermediate care nursery should be able to (1) monitor cardiopulmonary function; (2) assist with special procedures, such as lumbar punctures, endotracheal intubation, and umbilical vessel catheterization; and (3) perform emergency resuscitation. One member of the nursing staff is required on each shift for every three to four neonates who need intermediate care (6–7 hours care every 24 hours). Nursing staff in this area should be able to initiate, modify, or stop treatment when appropriate—even if a physician is not present—according to established protocols. If assisted ventilation is needed, persons who can intubate the trachea; change the pressure, flow, and frequency of mechanical ventilation; and decompress a pneumothorax by needle aspiration should be available. In these situations, it is appropriate to provide one professional nurse for each neonate. The professional activities of nurses with expanded roles should be under the direction of the unit's medical director.

Laboratory, radiology, and ultrasound technicians should be in-hospital or on call at all times to ensure that they are readily available when needed in the maternal-fetal and neonatal care areas. Respiratory therapists with special training in neonatal care should be in-hospital at all times. Social services personnel who can provide family counseling and advice should also be available. Special nutritional counseling is also required.

HOSPITALS PROVIDING LEVEL III SERVICES

Level III Medical Staff

The maternal-fetal medicine service should be directed by a full-time, board-certified obstetrician who is qualified by training, experience, or special competence certification in maternal-fetal medicine. The regional newborn intensive care unit should be directed by a full-time, board-certified pediatrician with special competence and, in most cases, subspecialty certification in neonatal medicine. As codirectors of the perinatal service, these physicians are responsible for maintenance of standards of patient care, development of the operating budget, equip-ment evaluation and purchase, planning and development of in-hos-pital as well as outreach educational programs, coordination of these elements, and evaluation of the effectiveness of perinatal care in the region. They should devote their time to patient care services, research, and teaching, as well as coordination with level I and II hospitals in the area.

Other neonatologists who practice in the facility need not be hospital-based, but they should have qualifications similar to those of the chief of service. One neonatologist should be provided for every six to ten patients in the continuing care, intermediate care, and inten-sive care areas. (A ratio of one physician in training [residents or fellows] to every four or five patients who require intensive care is ideal, but this is practical only in centers with a full complement of personnel.) A neonatologist should be available on a 24-hour basis for consultation.

Board-certified anesthesiologists with special training or experi-ence in maternal-fetal anesthesia should be in charge of perinatal anesthesia services. Personnel capable of administering obstetric, neo-natal, and pediatric anesthesia should be available at all times. Ultra-sound services should be available on a 24-hour basis. This diagnostic service should be under the direction of a physician who has a special interest in obstetric diagnoses and complications. Radiology services should be under the direction of a board-certified radiologist with special competence in pediatric radiology. Pediatric subspecialists, both surgical and medical, in cardiology, neurology, hematology, and genetics should be available for consultation. Consultant services in renal function, metabolism, endocrinology, gastroenterology-nutrition, hematology, infectious diseases, pulmonary medicine, immunology, and pharmacology are also needed. Pediatric surgical subspecialists, e.g., cardiovascular surgeons, plastic surgeons, and neurosurgeons, as well as orthopedic, ophthalmologic, urologic, and ear, nose and throat surgeons, should also be available for consultation and care. A pathologist with special competence in placental, fetal, and neonatal disease, also should be a member of the hospital staff.

Level III Nursing Staff

The supervisor of perinatal nursing services in hospitals providing level III care should have certification or advanced skills and training in perinatal nursing care. The supervisor should be assisted by an administrative coordinator responsible for schedules and staffing. Both neonatal and maternal-fetal services should have a head nurse who is responsible for the direct nursing care provided to patients on each service. The intermediate and intensive care nursery areas should also have a head nurse.

The nursing staff in the labor, delivery, and postpartum areas should have certification or advanced education and experience in the nursing management of both normal and high-risk laboring patients and their families. Nursing staff should further be experienced in handling obstetric and medical complications of pregnancy. It is essential to good patient care for nursing staff to be able to make adequate assessments of the patient's condition and progress in labor.

Recommended nurse/patient ratios in the special care nursery areas are suggested in Table 3–1. As training programs develop, some of these nurses may become neonatal nurse-clinicians.

SUPPORT PERSONNEL

In all facilities a blood bank technician should always be available for determining blood type, cross-matching blood, and performing Coombs' tests. Various other personnel are required to provide support services, but the intensity and level of sophistication of these services vary with the level of program development. For example, the hospital's infection control personnel should be responsible for surveillance of infections in mothers and neonates and for the development of an appropriate environmental control program (see Surveillance for Nosocomial Infection, Chapter 6).

At least one full-time medical social worker who has experience · with the socioeconomic and psychosocial problems of high-risk mothers and fetuses, sick neonates, and their families should be assigned to the maternal-fetal service; another should be assigned to the neonatal service.

A minimum of one registered perinatal dietitian/nutritionist should be available to plan diets to meet the special needs of high-risk mothers and neonates.

The hospital's engineering department should include air-conditioning, electronic, and mechanical engineers, as well as biomedical technicians, who are responsible for the safety and reliability of the equipment in the labor and delivery area and the special care nurseries.

Qualified personnel for support services, such as laboratory studies, x-ray, and ultrasound, should be available at all times. In level II and III facilities, these personnel should be in the hospital on a 24-hour basis.

Respiratory therapists or nurses with special training in the ventilation of sick neonates should be available to supervise the assisted ventilation of neonates with cardiopulmonary disease. One therapist is needed for each four neonates receiving assisted ventilation.

EDUCATION

In-Service and Continuing Education

The medical and nursing staffs of hospitals that provide perinatal care at any level should have at least one joint teaching session each month concerning maternal and neonatal health. These sessions should cover diagnosis and management of perinatal emergencies, as well as the management of routine problems. The staff of each unit should also have a monthly conference at which special patient care problems that arose during the month are presented and discussed. The chief or chiefs of service and the head nurse or nurses are responsible for this program of continuing education.

Medical and nursing staffs of hospitals that provide level I and II care should participate in formal courses and conferences sponsored by the regional perinatal resource center. The staff of the regional center should assist with the in-service programs of other hospitals in their region on a regular basis. Such assistance should include periodic visits to those hospitals, as well as timely consultation and participation in patient care. Periodic review of the quality of patient care should be a fundamental part of such a program. Regional center staff should be accessible for consultation at all times.

The regional center should have regularly scheduled conferences including, as a minimum, those in the following list:

1. Weekly conferences to review major perinatal illnesses of the past week and plan for anticipated perinatal problems
2. Monthly conferences to review perinatal statistics, the pathology related to all deaths, and significant surgical specimens
3. Weekly conferences to review current x-ray films and ultrasonography material
4. Administrative staff conferences to review procedures and policies
5. Teaching seminars on perinatal subjects for nursing and medical staffs

Perinatal Outreach Education

The coordinator of a perinatal outreach education program should be a registered nurse with advanced skills and experience in maternal-fetal or pediatric nursing, clinical experience in nursing management of mothers or neonates, and experience and preparation in teaching. This coordinator should be responsible for the development and management of the program. Responsibilities should include assessing needs, planning curricula, teaching, implementing an evaluation program, collecting and utilizing perinatal data, providing patient follow-up information to referring community personnel, writing reports, and maintaining informative working relationships with community personnel and outreach team members.

A maternal-fetal specialist, an obstetric nurse, a neonatologist, and a neonatal nurse are the essential members of the perinatal outreach team. Each member should be responsible for teaching, consulting with community professionals as needed, and maintaining communication with the coordinator and other team members. Other professionals, e.g., a social worker, a respiratory therapist, or a nutritionist, may be assigned to the perinatal outreach education team on a part-time basis.

Each regional perinatal care center is responsible for organizing an education program tailored to the identified needs of the perinatal health professionals employed in community institutions in its area. The program may include perinatal morbidity and mortality statistics, case presentations, progress reports of maternal and neonatal patients transported to the regional center, and a pertinent topic presentation.

These perinatal outreach meetings should be held at a routine time and place to allow for a continuity of communication among community professionals and regional center personnel. This facilitates the development of mutual trust among perinatal care providers.

Perinatal outreach activities have been characterized in part by their emphasis on a team approach. Therefore, a topic presentation with a clinical and patient focus often may include the medical and nursing perspectives. Professionals from other disciplines, e.g., social workers, nutritionists, respiratory therapists, or perinatal anesthesiologists, should be utilized as necessary to fulfill the identified educational needs of the area.

The perinatal outreach education program can be evaluated in part by the collection of perinatal morbidity and mortality data. Chart audits at community hospitals and clinics may also be useful.

RESOURCES AND RECOMMENDED READING

National Foundation–March of Dimes, Committee on Perinatal Health: Toward Improving the Outcome of Pregnancy: Recommendations for the regional development of maternal and perinatal health services. National Foundation–March of Dimes, White Plains, NY, 1977

Nurses Association of the American College of Obstetricians and Gynecologists: Nurse Providers of Neonatal Intensive Care: Guidelines for educational development and practice. Washington, DC, NAACOG, 1982

Nurses Association of the American College of Obstetricians and Gynecologists: Obstetric-Gynecologic Nurse Practitioner: Role Definition, Role Description, Guidelines for Educational Development. Washington, DC, NAACOG, 1979

Nurses Association of the American College of Obstetricians and Gynecologists: Standards for Obstetric, Gynecologic, and Neonatal Nursing, 2 ed. Washington, DC, NAACOG, 1981 chapter

4
Perinatal Care Services

Perinatal care directly affects the outcome of pregnancy. A comprehensive program involves an integrated approach to medical care and psychosocial support rendered throughout pregnancy and the perinatal period, including risk assessment, serial surveillance, prenatal education, utilization of specialized skills and technology, observation of the mother and neonate, preparation for discharge, and follow-up during the postpartum period. To achieve optimal results, a comprehensive program should focus on the delivery of safe, high-quality care while at the same time recognizing pregnancy and childbirth as a family experience.

Most patients are eager to participate in decisions that affect their pregnancy. These patients usually are well-informed and motivated, health conscious, and receptive to professional guidance. Patients should be encouraged to express their preferences regarding decisions that relate to procedures performed during the childbirth process, such as invasive monitoring, perineal preparation, episiotomy, and enema. They may also express their opinions concerning intrapartum medications, methods of pain relief, and length of hospital stay.

Obstetric care has become more flexible, and more options are available to women. These include alternatives regarding birthing environments, the presence of a supporting person during labor and delivery, bonding, and rooming-in. Specific hospital policies, especially those pertaining to a childbirth coach, the presence of the father and other family members at labor and delivery and visiting should be explained to the patient well in advance of the estimated date of confinement.

Families and professionals should interact throughout the antepartum, intrapartum, postpartum and neonatal periods in order to develop mutual respect and trust and to enhance care.

FAMILY-CENTERED CARE

A fundamental goal of maternal and newborn care is to foster parent-newborn-family relationships. The concept of family-centered care should be integrated into every aspect of perinatal services. The document *Family-Centered Maternity/Newborn Care in Hospitals* describes how the various members of the health care team can work together in achieving a family-centered approach to the care provided.

The family nucleus should be identified early in the antepartum period so that family participation can be as complete as possible. Participation of the support person throughout the intrapartum and postpartum periods should be clearly understood by all persons involved. The support person should be prepared to assume his or her appropriate role during labor, and the degree of involvement should be clearly defined.

Health care professionals assume an important role in this approach to care. The process should begin during the first prenatal visit with a review of the parents' attitudes toward the pregnancy, family life, child care practices, stresses in the mother's environment, support systems, and interest in childbirth education classes. It continues throughout the perinatal period in both the ambulatory and hospital settings.

ANTEPARTUM CARE

To achieve the best possible pregnancy outcome, every woman should have a comprehensive program of antepartum care that begins as early as possible in the first trimester of pregnancy. Early diagnosis of pregnancy is an important factor in establishing a management plan appropriate to the individual. There are three main components of antepartum care: (1) serial surveillance, which begins with a comprehensive history and physical examination to identify risk factors or abnormalities and to establish the date of confinement; (2) patient education to foster optimal health, good dietary habits, and proper hygiene; and (3) appropriate psychosocial support.

Serial Surveillance

Antepartum care begins with the first prenatal visit when the important physician-patient relationship begins. At this time, an obstetric data base should be established; it should contain information derived from a comprehensive health history, including information regarding the last menstrual period, the current pregnancy, a review of past obstetric outcome, and medical, family, and social history; dietary assessment (see Chapter 7); physical examination; estimated date of confinement; laboratory procedures; and risk assessment. Medical conditions affect pregnancy outcome (see Risk Assessment, this chapter). Early identification of such conditions to establish an appropriate treatment plan, to maintain rigid surveillance, and to plan for delivery can minimize maternal and neonatal morbidity.

History

The health history should include a review of past pregnancies: fullterm or premature deliveries, spontaneous and induced abortions, health status of living children, spacing of previous pregnancies, length of each gestation, route of delivery, sex and weight of the newborn, Rho(D) immune globulin (RhIG) administration with previous pregnancies, and any complications, particularly those resulting in fetal or neonatal deaths.

In addition, important information that helps identify the patient at risk, such as alcohol consumption, cigarette smoking, and exposure to radiation, should be obtained (see Risk Assessment, this chapter). The list of environmental hazards for which there is enough information to make clinical recommendations is limited. Any time there is a question of exposure to possible teratogenic agents, expert consultation and counseling may be helpful.

The history should also include questions about susceptibility to immunizable diseases, immunizations received, and recent exposures to acute communicable diseases. Administration of some vaccines during pregnancy is contraindicated; fortunately, immunization of women during pregnancy is necessary only rarely. If a pregnant woman has been exposed recently or is likely to be exposed to a specific immunizable disease, current information about risks of the disease and the risks and benefits of vaccine administration should be evaluated before a course of action is selected (see Table 6–2).

The family history should be thorough, including information on metabolic disorders, cardiovascular disease, malignancy, congenital abnormalities, mental retardation, and multiple births. It is important to obtain a family history of congenital anomalies to enable identification of the fetus at risk for an inherited disease. The previous birth of a child with congenital anomalies demands a detailed history of the particulars in anticipation of the need for prenatal genetic counseling and studies (see Antenatal Detection of Genetic Disorders, Chapter 10). A history of repeated midtrimester losses or premature delivery should alert the physician and parents to the significant risk of recurrence and the possible need for consultative services. It should also be remembered that women of high parity are at increased risk for puerperal hemorrhage, multiple gestation, and placenta previa.

The social history should include the patient's occupation and work environment, ethnic origin, educational background, and lifestyle.

Establishment of the Expected Date of Confinement

The expected date of confinement is best determined in a patient who begins receiving care early in pregnancy and receives regular prenatal care. Problems such as intrauterine growth retardation, premature labor, and postterm pregnancy cannot be detected or managed effectively when accurate information is not available.

Accuracy of the expected date of confinement is confirmed by ascertaining the regularity, duration, and individual character of the menstrual cycle, including changes in bleeding patterns. Errors in dating pregnancy can result from failure to consider menstrual irregularities, longer-than-average cycle lengths, recent use of oral contraceptive steroids, and the possibility that what appeared to be the last menstrual period was actually implantation bleeding.

Physical Examination

Every woman should receive a complete physical examination that includes an evaluation of the height, weight, blood pressure, head, neck, breasts, heart, lungs, abdomen, pelvis, rectum, extremities, and current nutritional status. The size and shape of the uterus and adnexal areas, and the configuration and capacity of the bony pelvis should be evaluated with bimanual examination and properly recorded.

Early pregnancy is the most accurate time to correlate uterine size and duration of gestation. The uterus is usually a pelvic organ until the 12th week of gestation. At midpregnancy (20 weeks' gestation), it usually reaches the umbilicus. Between the 18th and 34th week, uterine height, as measured by calipers or a tape in centimeters from the top of the symphysis pubis to the top of the uterine fundus, approximates the gestational age (in weeks). At 18–20 weeks' gestation, fetal heart tones can be heard with a fetoscope, although they may be heard with a Doppler device as early as 10–12 weeks' gestation. With real-time ultrasonography, fetal heart activity can be seen as soon as 3–4 weeks after the first missed period.

Laboratory Tests

Those laboratory tests that should be performed as early in pregnancy as possible include the following:

Hemoglobin or hematocrit levels
Urinalysis for protein and glucose
Blood group and Rh type
Irregular antibody screen
Rubella antibody titer (if previous immunity not determined)
Cervical cytology
Serologic testing for syphilis

The need for additional laboratory evaluations should be determined by historical factors or unusual findings derived from the history and physical examination. The ethnic, racial, and social origins of the patient also may dictate the need for special testing, such as urine culture, cervical culture for gonorrhea, plasma glucose determination, sickle cell test, and skin test for tuberculosis. (See Specific Infectious Problems during Pregnancy and Management of the Newborn, Chapter 6, for further information regarding testing for syphilis, gonorrhea, and tuberculosis.)

Early in the third trimester, an additional test should be done to determine hemoglobin or hematocrit level. A repeat test for venereal diseases should be performed if the patient belongs to a high-risk population. At some time during the patient's antepartum course, it may be appropriate to repeat an irregular antibody screen. Unsensitized Rh-negative patients should have repeat antibody tests at about 28, 32, and 36 weeks' gestation. All abnormal values require work-up and serial surveillance.

Prophylactic administration of RhIG during the antepartum and postpartum periods has been helpful in further reducing the incidence of Rho(D) isoimmunization. A national recommendation for routine administration of RhIG has not been made at this time, however. When antepartum prophylaxis is elected by the physician and patient, 300 μg RhIG should be administered intramuscularly at 28–32 weeks' gestation to a nonisoimmunized Rho(D)-negative woman when the father is known to be Rho(D)-positive. It is important to remember that repeat administration is necessary at delivery if the newborn is Rh-positive.

Subsequent Visits

The frequency of return visits should be determined by the woman's individual needs and risk assessment. Generally, a woman with an uncomplicated pregnancy should be seen every 4 weeks for the first 28 weeks of pregnancy, every 2–3 weeks until 36 weeks' gestation, and weekly thereafter, although flexibility is desirable. Women with medical or obstetric problems require closer surveillance at intervals determined by the nature and severity of the problems.

At each follow-up visit, the patient should be given an opportunity to ask questions about her pregnancy or comment on changes she has noted. During each visit, blood pressure, weight, uterine size, and, when appropriate, fetal presentation and heart rate, should be assessed. Urinalysis should be performed to detect protein and glucose. Any change in the pregnancy risk assessment should be recorded after each evaluation, and an appropriate management plan outlined.

Risk Assessment

Continual risk assessment should be a standard part of antenatal care. For most effective clinical use, risk assessment instruments must be simple, rapid, and easy to interpret.

Identification of the high-risk patient is critical to minimize maternal and neonatal morbidity and mortality. As illustrated in Figure 4–1, there is ample evidence to show that known risk factors can be used to identify high-risk patients early in the antenatal course, as well as intrapartally. Approximately 20% of pregnant women can be identified prenatally to be at risk, accounting for 55% of poor pregnancy outcomes. In addition, 5–10% of pregnant women can be identified to be at risk for the first time during labor, resulting in 20–25% of poor pregnancy outcomes. Thus, a total of 25–30% of pregnant women who are identified to be at risk during either the antepartum or intrapartum periods result in 75–80% of poor pregnancy outcomes. It is important to recognize, however, that 20% of perinatal morbidity and mortality will arise from the group without identifiable risks.

Risk assessment is influenced by medical and obstetric considerations, as well as the patient's lifestyle and environmental factors. Maternal cigarette smoking and low birth weight are known to be related. Excessive alcohol consumption has been associated with fetal alcohol syndrome, and even seemingly moderate consumption of alcohol is now implicated as problematic by dysmorphologists. Although abdominal and pelvic exposure of less than 5 rad has not been asso-

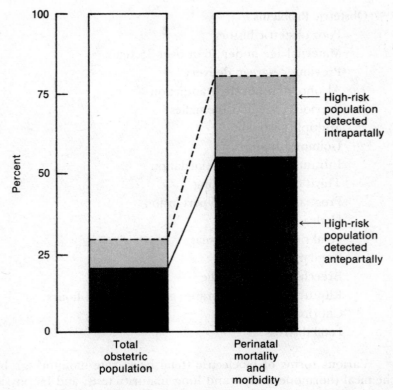

Fig. 4–1. *High-risk pregnancy outcome. (Ryan GM Jr (ed): Ambulatory Care in Obstetrics and Gynecology. New York, Grune & Stratton, 1980)*

ciated with identifiable biologic injuries to the fetus, higher exposures may be harmful. The following is a partial list of high-risk factors, derived from the history or physical examination, that increase pregnancy risks and that might necessitate further evaluation, consultation, or referral:

Medical Problems

    Cardiovascular, renal, collagen, pulmonary, infectious, liver, and venereal diseases

    Chronic urinary tract infections

    Maternal viral, bacterial, and protozoan infections

    Diabetes mellitus

    Severe anemia

    Isoimmune thrombocytopenia

    Convulsive disorders

Obstetric Problems
Poor obstetric history
Maternal age under 16 or over 35 years
Previous cesarean delivery
Alcohol or other drug addiction
Previous cogenital anomalies
Multiple gestation
Isoimmunization
Intrauterine growth retardation
Third trimester bleeding
Pregnancy-induced hypertension
Hydramnios
Fetal cardiac arrhythmias
Prematurity
Breech or transverse lie
Rupture of the membranes greater than 24 hours
Chorioamnionitis
Fetal distress

Various forms of bioelectric (fetal heart rate monitoring), bio-chemical (hormone assays) and lung maturity tests, and biophysical (ultrasound) tests should be available for patients when risk factors indicate their need. When the availability of these technologic resources is limited, appropriate arrangements should be made for a regional-ized network to provide access to facilities with such resources.

Gestational age is an important factor in the management of pregnancy, particularly in the presence of high-risk factors when appropriately timed intervention may be necessary. The criteria sug-gested for assessing fetal maturity prior to elective repeat cesarean delivery and elective induction of labor (see page 66) may be useful guidelines for confirming gestational age in all pregnancies. The appropriate timing of intervention should take into account this infor-mation along with other clinical evaluations and laboratory data. When a pregnancy to be terminated is less than 39 weeks' (273 days') gestation amniotic fluid analysis for the determination of lecithin/sphingomyelin (L/S) ratio or phosphatidylglycerol may provide satisfactory evidence of fetal lung maturity.

In many instances, special obstetric problems require a multidis-ciplinary approach. To ensure appropriate care at the time of delivery, the obstetrician should inform the pediatrician when there is a significant risk factor for the neonate. In all pregnancies, especially high-risk pregnancies, it is important that the pediatrician meet with the couple and discuss plans for neonatal evaluation and management. Some high-risk conditions may require transport of the fetus in utero (maternal-fetal transport), which in most circumstances is preferable to transport of a high-risk neonate.

Premature rupture of the membranes or labor is the leading cause of perinatal mortality in the United States. Despite extensive investigations, it remains a problem of early risk recognition, diagnosis, and treatment.

The obstetric or gynecologic history may provide some important clues to the diagnosis. A history of preterm deliveries, diethylstilbestrol (DES) exposure, heavy smoking, hypertension, chronic glomerulonephritis or pyelonephritis, or other chronic medical disorders have been implicated. A history of dilation and curettage (D&C) in the early teenage years; suction curettage, dilation, and evacuation for interruption of pregnancy; or cone biopsy have been associated with cervical incompetence. A history of progressively earlier second trimester deliveries without labor is consistent with, but not diagnostic of, cervical incompetence. Premature cervical dilation may be signaled by pelvic pressure, urinary frequency, watery vaginal discharge, cramps similar to menstrual cramps, low backache, vaginal bleeding, or uterine contractions. A high index of suspicion for premature labor, based on the history, dictates more intensive surveillance, which may lead to early diagnosis and intervention by either stopping labor, using cervical cerclage, administering drugs that influence lung maturity, or monitoring the course of labor to decrease asphyxia. Simple solutions cannot be offered for these problems, but certain risks can be identified, needs anticipated, and cooperative regional solutions provided.

A pregnancy that goes beyond term requires special attention. For a small but significant number of fetuses, prolonged pregnancy increases the risk of chronic intrauterine asphyxia, meconium aspiration, long-term neurologic handicap, and, occasionally, death. Such fetuses stand to benefit appreciably from antenatal care that includes early pregnancy dating, sizing and growth measurements, and the application of modern technology for assessment of fetal well-being. Fetal surveillance will identify for delivery those postterm fetuses who might be compromised by remaining in utero, while providing reassurance for the majority of patients whose fetuses are not at risk and whose pregnancies can be continued under surveillance.

With an awareness of the conditions that increase fetal risk, the final major decision of good antepartum care can be made; namely, the selection of the health care facility that can best meet the needs of the parturient and her child.

Patient Information

The physician and others providing health care should discuss the proposed plan of antepartum care with the patient. The discussion should include an explanation of the kind of care that is provided in the office, necessary laboratory studies, the expected course of the pregnancy, signs and symptoms to be reported to the physician (such as rupture of the membranes), the timing of subsequent visits, proper diet and health habits, educational programs available, options for intrapartum care, hospital protocols concerning family participation, and the general plans for hospital admission, labor, and delivery. The roles of various members of the health care team, office policies (including emergency coverage), and alternate physician coverage should also be explained. Specific information regarding costs should be provided.

Early in the third trimester, plans for hospital admission, labor, and delivery should be reviewed and information provided on what to do when labor begins, when the membranes rupture, or if bleeding occurs. Analgesic and anesthetic options should be discussed. Because a general anesthetic may be required for delivery, the patient should be advised of the hazards of ingesting food or fluid after the onset of labor. Aspects of newborn care, including circumcision of male neonates should be discussed.

Prenatal Education

The importance of prenatal education cannot be overemphasized. Ideally, education should begin prior to conception, preferably as a part of adolescent health care, since organogenesis is usually complete before the first prenatal visit. The months of pregnancy present an opportunity for health professionals to take advantage of the woman's motivation to share in the responsibility of health education and to do what is best for her baby. Suggested guidelines for preconceptual care are shown in Appendix C.

The physician should see that the woman is provided with information about nutrition. Smoking and excessive alcohol consumption should be discouraged. The patient should understand that moderate daily exercise is an important component of healthy pregnancy, but that a sensation of fatigue suggests overdoing. Pregnancy is not the time for competitive or dangerous sports or acquisition of new athletic skills. It is a time, however, for moderate exercise, such as walking, swimming, golf, and perhaps tennis. Jogging in moderation is permissible as long as the patient avoids overheating, dehydration, discomfort, and fatigue.

Childbirth Education

Patients should be referred to appropriate educational literature and urged to attend childbirth education classes. Such educational programs may be offered by the hospital or community agencies or groups and ideally should be conducted by personnel qualified to teach childbirth education. Participation of physicians and hospital obstetric nurses in educational programs is desirable to ensure continuity of care and consistency of instruction.

Childbirth education classes provide an excellent opportunity for women to learn specific information relating to the childbirth experience. Families should be encouraged to participate in childbirth education programs. Family members who have been adequately prepared can have a favorable and lasting influence on the mother, the neonate, and, ultimately, the family unit.

Following is a list of some of the topics included in a childbirth education class:

Anatomy and physiology of reproduction

Physiologic and psychological changes of pregnancy

Care during pregnancy

Nutritional needs

Teratogenic and other risks

Danger signs

Fetal growth and development

Role of the prospective father and siblings

Breathing and relaxation exercises

Options for obstetric anesthesia and analgesia

Signs of approaching labor

Stages of labor

Childbirth alternatives, cesarean delivery, or vaginal delivery after previous cesarean delivery

Breast-feeding techniques

Care of the neonate

Parenting skills

Family relationships
Subsequent family planning

Psychosocial Support

Pregnancy is a major event in a woman's life. It is a time in which the family is "expected" to be happy. However, pregnancy is a profound emotional experience. Conflicts may arise over involvement of grandparents, family life, expectations, and new responsibilities. An atmosphere of acceptance allows families to communicate their feelings. Group encounters, such as childbirth classes and antepartum breastfeeding seminars, may be helpful. On occasion, referral to appropriate psychological or psychiatric specialists may be necessary.

INTRAPARTUM CARE: LABOR AND DELIVERY

A woman should approach the unique experience of labor and delivery with a sense of confidence and trust in her antepartum preparation, in the skill and knowledge of her physician, and in a well-equipped hospital with a knowledgeable and experienced staff. Childbirth is a unique family experience, and the obstetric staff should strive to make the patient and the father or other supporting persons comfortable and to keep them informed. The father or other supporting persons may be encouraged to stay with the patient during labor and delivery in accordance with hospital policies.

In large measure, the patient's and family's perception of the intrapartum experience is influenced by information provided during the antepartum period, particularly in regard to the normal physiologic processes occurring within both mother and fetus. The father or supporting person puts into practice the principles that were learned regarding the conduct of labor. Mutual benefit can be derived from the supportive role of the father. Physical contact of the newborn with the parents in the delivery room may enhance future relationships, and hospital personnel should be encouraged to support the desire of the family to be together and, where feasible, to facilitate family interaction.

Intrapartum care should be both personalized and comprehensive. Since a significant proportion of patients ultimately attain high-risk status because of intrapartum complications, continuous surveillance of the mother and fetus is essential.

The hospital setting provides the safest atmosphere for the mother, fetus, and neonate during labor, delivery, and the postpartum period. Birth centers that are within the hospital complex and function under the protocols of the department of obstetrics and gynecology provide safeguards to ensure safety. Scientific methodology to investigate adequately the outcome of normal deliveries has been problematic, as documented in a study done by the National Academy of Sciences. Until scientific studies are available to evaluate safety and outcome in free-standing centers, the use of such centers cannot be encouraged. There may be exceptional geographically isolated situations, however, where special programs are necessary.

Admission Procedures, Medical Records, and Patient Consent Forms

At 36 weeks' gestation (or earlier, if indicated), the patient's prenatal care record should be available in the labor registration area. When the patient is admitted for labor and delivery, her prenatal care record should be reviewed (see Antepartum Care, this chapter); pertinent information from this record should be recorded on the admission note, e.g., blood group and Rh type, irregular antibody detection, serology, and other diagnostic tests and therapeutic measures. The nursing admission note should include (1) the patient's name, (2) reason for admission, (3) date and time of patient's arrival and notification of physician, and (4) time seen by the physician.

Patients in labor, with premature rupture of the membranes, or with vaginal bleeding should be admitted directly to the labor and delivery suite. Occasionally, obstetric patients who are not in labor but who require special intensive care also may be admitted to this area. The admission of a patient in prodromal labor with no complications may be deferred, and she may be allowed to ambulate or wait in a more casual, comfortable area. Patients suspected of having a transmissible infection, discharging skin lesions, diarrhea, or purulent vaginal discharge should be admitted to a specific labor, delivery, and recovery area where isolation techniques can be used according to established hospital policy (see also Chapter 6).

The evaluation of a patient who has had a recent examination and who is not at high risk may be restricted to a pertinent history. Attention should be focused on the onset of contractions, status of the membranes, bleeding, fetal activity, history of allergies, time and content of last ingestion, and the use of any medication.

The admitting physical examination should include the patient's blood pressure, pulse, and temperature. The fetal position, presentation, and heart rate, as well as the frequency, duration, and quality of the uterine contractions, should be recorded. The degree of cervical dilation, effacement, status of the membranes, or any unusual bleeding should be noted prior to the initial pelvic examination. The responsible physician must be notified immediately if any complications are determined so that the patient's condition may be promptly evaluated. A urine sample should be tested to determine the presence of protein and glucose.

The fetal heart rate should be determined and recorded as soon as the patient arrives in the admitting area so that a baseline measurement will be available should fetal distress be suspected. When there are no complications or contraindications, trained nursing personnel may perform the initial pelvic examination. The physician responsible for the patient's care should be informed of her status so that a decision can be made regarding further management. If anesthesia other than local or pudendal is anticipated or desired, anesthesia personnel should be informed soon after the patient's admission. The results of the patient examination should be noted on the record, and diagnostic and therapeutic orders, as well as any necessary consent forms, should be signed and included with the record.

Departmental policies and physician preference concerning admission procedures, such as shaving of the pubic and perineal hair, enemas, showers, tie-in-the-back gowns, intravenous lines, abdominal belts or electronic fetal monitoring, and ambulatory restrictions, should take into account the patient's needs and preferences. In addition, the use of drugs for analgesia and anesthesia during labor should depend on the needs and desires of the patient and on the judgment of the attending physician. Access to the intravascular space is necessary for administration of drugs, fluids, or blood. A line to the intravascular space should be established, preferably through a large bore in-dwelling plastic catheter, for women who will or who may require a general (inhalation or induction) anesthetic.

Patients who have had no prenatal care should undergo a complete history and physical examination, blood count, blood typing and Rh determination, and urine testing upon admission. A patient who has not had an orientation visit to the labor and delivery area as a part of childbirth education or who is unfamiliar with monitoring techniques that might be used during labor should be given a careful explanation of what will happen during labor.

Pain Relief During Labor and Delivery

Control of discomfort and pain during labor and delivery is more than providing personal comfort to the mother; it is a necessary part of good obstetric practice. Pain can be controlled by pharmacologic means or through childbirth education and preparation that teaches the patient how to cope with the discomfort of labor and delivery. The choice and availability of analgesic and anesthetic techniques are influenced by the experience and training of the anesthetist, by the circumstances of labor and delivery, and by the personal preferences of the obstetrician and the patient.

Of the various pharmacologic methods used for pain relief during labor and delivery, continuous lumbar epidural analgesia is the most effective and least depressant; furthermore, it allows for an alert, participating mother. Narcotics and inhalation analgesia provide varying degrees of pain relief and can be used safely but are potentially depressant to both mother and fetus. Barbiturates, tranquilizers, and scopolamine have no analgesic qualities and are also potentially depressant. At the time of delivery, local infiltration and pudendal block are safe techniques with or without an inhalation analgesic supplement; however, they do not provide total pain relief and thus are not sufficient for all vaginal births. Spinal anesthesia can provide adequate pain relief and muscle relaxation for nearly all vaginal births. Unlike the continuous lumbar epidural, however, spinal anesthesia is useful only at the time of birth, and additional measures are required for pain control during the first stage of labor. Most importantly, general anesthesia is rarely necessary for vaginal births and should be used only for specific indications.

For the uncomplicated cesarean delivery, properly administered general or regional anesthesia is effective and has little adverse effect on the newborn. However, because of the risks to the mother associated with intubation and the occasional difficulty of aspiration, regional analgesia may be the safer technique and should be available to all parturients. The advantages and disadvantages of both techniques should be discussed as completely as possible.

If properly chosen and administered, anesthesia or analgesia has little or no effect on the physiologic status of the neonate. At present, there are no long-term studies available that determine if subtle findings in neonatal neurobehavior associated with the administration of anesthesia or analgesia to the woman in labor have a significant correlation with the child's later mental and neurologic development.

Since the safety of obstetric anesthesia depends principally on the skill of the anesthetist, and since obstetric anesthesia must be considered emergency anesthesia, it demands a competence of personnel and availability of equipment similar to or greater than that required for elective procedures. Obstetricians, house officers, nurse-anesthetists, and nonphysician personnel are seldom fully competent in all forms of inhalation, intravenous, local, regional, and conduction block anesthesia. It is the responsibility of the director of anesthesia services to review the qualifications and competence of each individual who is to provide anesthesia or analgesia and to determine which agents and techniques he or she may use. The director of anesthesia services, with the approval of the medical staff, should develop and enforce written policies regarding provision of obstetric anesthesia, i.e., who may do specific procedures and under what circumstances. The obstetric patient should be anesthetized only when a qualified physician is immediately available to supervise the labor and to deal with any complication that may arise.

An obstetrician trained in the appropriate methods of anesthesia administration may administer the anesthesia if privileges for these procedures have been granted by the obstetric and anesthesia departments. However, it is preferable for an anesthesiologist or anesthetist to provide this care so the obstetrician may devote undivided attention to the delivery. All obstetricians should be trained in the use of infiltration anesthesia. When any type of regional anesthesia is administered, the patient should be monitored by a qualified member of the health care team.

Management of Labor

Patients Without Identifiable Risks

It is important to recognize that 20% of perinatal morbidity and mortality will arise during the intrapartum period from the group of patients who have had no complications during their pregnancies and who are considered "normal." Therefore, basic standards of care should be maintained in this group of patients, i.e., those without identifiable risks, in order to minimize problems of an unpredictable nature that may be encountered.

After the patient in labor has been admitted and her status initially evaluated, ongoing intrapartum surveillance is necessary, although the degree and method required will vary according to predetermined risk factors. For each shift she is in the labor and delivery area, the patient should be introduced to the nurse responsible for her care. A designated member of the obstetric team should be responsible for observing the patient, following the progress of labor, and recording the patient's vital signs and fetal heart rate on the labor record. The physician responsible for the patient's care should be kept informed of her progress and notified immediately of any abnormality. The patient may be permitted to ambulate with the knowledge and consent of the attending physician. General care during labor should provide optimal patient comfort in additional to optimal fetal and maternal safety.

For the patient without identifiable risks, assessment of the quality of uterine contractions, in conjunction with a pelvic examination, should be adequate to detect evidence of any abnormality and to monitor the progress of labor. Fetal heart rate also should be evaluated immediately after rupture of the membranes. The patient's temperature and pulse should be recorded every 4 hours, and more often if indicated. Maternal blood pressure should be taken and recorded every hour during labor and immediately prior to delivery. The patient should be encouraged to void every 3 hours during labor. The amount of fluid intake and output should be recorded. The fetal heart rate should be recorded at least every 30 minutes immediately following a uterine contraction in the first stage of labor and at no more than 15-minute intervals in the second stage of labor until preparation for delivery. Any new significant symptom or sign (e.g., excessive vaginal bleeding or pain, or meconium-stained amniotic fluid) should be evaluated by the physician.

Patients should not take anything by mouth during labor except for small sips of water or preparations to moisten the mouth and lips. Hydration and nourishment during long labors should be provided via intravenous fluids; this measure also minimizes acidosis and electrolyte imbalance.

Because aspiration continues to be a leading cause of anesthetic-related maternal mortality and because aspiration of acidic (pH<2.5) gastric contents is more harmful than less acidic gastric contents, the prophylactic administration of an antacid before general anesthesia seems appropriate. Animal studies indicate that particulate antacids may be harmful if aspirated; therefore, a clear antacid, such as 0.03 M sodium citrate or a similar preparation, may be a safer choice.

Vaginal examinations should be kept to a minimum and conducted with careful attention to use of a clean technique. Cleansing of the perineum with an antiseptic like providone-iodine or use of a sterile lubricant may decrease potential contamination and discomfort from the examination.

All hospitals with labor and delivery services should have the capability of continuous electronic fetal monitoring, although routine use of electronic fetal monitoring for all patients is not required. Uterine contractions can be assessed by the traditional method of placing the hand on the abdomen. An external abdominal transducer with an electronic tracing can accurately document the frequency of uterine contractions and their temporal relation to periodic fetal heart rate changes, thus permitting screening of the fetus who may be in distress.

High-Risk Patients

Continuous electronic monitoring should be used for patients identified as high-risk. External electronic monitoring allows accurate and close scrutiny of the fetal heart rate as it changes in relation to contractions. It permits detection of fetal heart rate patterns that have ominous significance, e.g., late decelerations and severe variable deceleration patterns. Directly applied fetal electrodes can be more accurate in evaluating beat-to-beat variability and may clarify the presence of fetal distress. When electronic fetal heart rate monitoring is used, the physician and obstetric personnel responsible for the patient should be qualified to identify and interpret abnormalities. Consultation with qualified physicians should be sought when abnormalities cannot be adequately interpreted by the staff responsible for the patient. Internal uterine monitoring provides important information regarding the quantity and quality of contractions, but it has the potential of introducing maternal or fetal infection and should not be used routinely (see Intrauterine Pressure and Fetal Monitoring, Chapter 6).

Notation on the monitoring strip of such items as the patient's position in the bed, cervical status, oxygen or drug administration, hypertension or hypotension, fever, amniotomy, color of the amniotic fluid, and Valsalva efforts provides a detailed and graphic documentation of the course of events during labor. Abnormal findings should be described and interpreted. Each recording should include the patient's name, hospital number, date and time of admission and delivery, and other data required for medical records. All tracings should be stored and readily retrievable.

Assessment of the fetal blood pH can clarify suspicious or confusing fetal heart rate patterns and confirm suspected fetal acidosis. This procedure should be performed on reliable and frequently calibrated equipment by personnel trained to identify and interpret abnormalities.

Medical Induction and Augmentation of Labor

Induction or augmentation of labor with oxytocin should be initiated only after the responsible physician has determined that it is beneficial to the mother or fetus. Consultation should be obtained prior to infusion when the physician does not have full obstetric privileges.

Each hospital's department of obstetrics and gynecology should determine the indications for induction and augmentation of labor and establish a protocol for the preparation and administration of the oxytocic solution.

Amniotomy has been used to induce and augment labor. Rupturing the membranes allows the physician to examine amniotic fluid for blood or meconium, to place a fetal scalp electrode or intrauterine catheter, or to obtain fetal scalp blood. However, the risks of amniotomy, such as cord prolapse and increased risk of chorioamnionitis, should be kept in mind.

Management of Delivery

Specific preparation for delivery should be started at a time dictated by the patient's parity, labor progress, fetal presentation, labor complications, and anesthesia management. When delivery is imminent, the patient should not be left unattended. At least one member of the nursing staff should be present in the delivery room throughout the delivery. Under no circumstances should any attempt be made to delay the birth by physical restraint or anesthesia.

For a patient without identifiable risks, delivery may be conducted in birthing rooms (see Chapter 2). However, the standards of care for the mother and the neonate that apply in a traditional setting also apply in a birthing room.

In those circumstances in which the delivery room is selected or indicated, the patient should be moved to the delivery table after transfer to the delivery room. A subarachnoid lumbar block anesthesia, if elected, may be administered at this time. After an appropriate interval for proper distribution of the anesthetic agent in the cerebrospinal fluid (CSF), the patient is positioned in preparation for delivery. Although the lithotomy position is generally used for vaginal delivery in the United States, many physicians prefer the lateral position or partial sitting position. Regardless of the position employed, positioning of the patient must be conducted safely with regard to the anesthesia involved.

When the patient has been positioned, she should be prepared for delivery. If a pudendal block or local perineal block anesthesia is used, it should be administered at this time.

Although episiotomy is indicated under certain circumstances (e.g., in the presence of a firm perineum that could tear during delivery, when operative vaginal delivery is required, or when there is a risk of trauma to the fetal head), its routine use is not recommended.

During delivery, the maternal blood pressure and pulse should be evaluated every 10 minutes and recorded. If electronic fetal monitoring has not been used or has been discontinued, the fetal heart rate should be evaluated by ascultation every 10 minutes. Maternal blood pressure and pulse should be evaluated upon delivery and reevaluated at 15-minute intervals (or more frequently) until the patient's condition has stabilized.

Assessment of Fetal Maturity Prior to Repeat Cesarean Delivery or Elective Induction of Labor

The assessment of fetal maturity is an important consideration in determining the timing of a repeat cesarean delivery or elective induction of labor. Fetal maturity can be assumed if at least two of the following clinical criteria for estimating gestational age are supported by at least one of the following laboratory determinations:

CLINICAL CRITERIA

1. Thirty-nine weeks have elapsed since the last menstrual period of a patient with normal menstrual cycles and no immediate antecedent use of oral contraceptives.
2. Fetal heart tones have been documented for 20 weeks by non-electric fetoscope.
3. Uterine size has been established by pelvic examination prior to 16 weeks' gestation.

LABORATORY DETERMINATIONS

1. Thirty-seven weeks have elapsed since a positive serum human chorionic gonadotropin (hCG) pregnancy test, or
2. Ultrasound
   a. Measurement based on the crown rump length obtained between 6 and 14 weeks' gestation, or
   b. Measurement based on the biparietal diameter obtained before 20 weeks' gestation.

If these criteria are not met, amniotic fluid analysis for lecithin/sphingomyelin (L/S) ratio or phosphatidylglycerol may provide satisfactory evidence of fetal lung maturity.

When there is no evidence of fetal lung maturity, it is a reasonable option to allow a patient with no contraindications to go into labor.

Repeat cesarean delivery does not necessarily constitute a high-risk situation for the neonate. Because the duties of the surgical team may preclude their caring for a distressed neonate, however, another qualified person should be present in the delivery room to care for the neonate.

Vaginal Delivery After Cesarean Childbirth

There has been increasing interest in permitting a trial of labor and vaginal delivery for a pregnant woman who has had a previous cesarean delivery. Suggested guidelines for those physicians and patients who wish to attempt vaginal delivery under these circumstances are available from the American College of Obstetricians and Gynecologists.

Assessment and Care of the Neonate in the Delivery Room

The first minutes of life may determine the quality of that life. Prompt, organized, and skilled response to emergencies in this period requires that institutions delivering maternal-fetal care have written policies delineating responsibility for immediate newborn care, resuscitation, selection and maintenance of necessary equipment, and training of personnel in proper techniques.

The individual who delivers the neonate is responsible for the immediate postdelivery care of the newborn until another person assumes this duty. Routine care of the healthy newborn may be delegated to appropriately trained nurses.

Recognition and immediate resuscitation of the distressed neonate requires an organized plan of action and immediate availability of qualified personnel and equipment. Planning for the provision of such services and equipment should be carried out jointly by the directors of the departments of obstetrics, anesthesia, and pediatrics, with the approval of the medical staff. A physician should be designated to assume primary responsibility for initiating, supervising, and reviewing the plan for management of depressed neonates in the delivery room. The following should be considered in this plan:

1. A list of maternal and fetal complications that require the presence in the delivery room of someone specifically qualified in newborn resuscitation should be developed. A sample list of high-risk conditions appears in Appendix D.

2. Responsibility for identification and resuscitation of distressed neonates should be assigned to an individual who is both specifically trained and immediately available in the hospital at all times. This may be a physician or an appropriately supervised nurse-midwife,

labor and delivery nurse, nurse-anesthetist, nursery nurse, or respiratory therapist.

3. Individuals qualified to perform neonatal resuscitation should demonstrate
   a. Skills in rapid and accurate evaluation of the newborn condition, including Apgar scoring.
   b. Knowledge of the pathogenesis and causes of a low Apgar score (asphyxia, drugs, hypovolemia, trauma, anomalies, and infection), as well as specific indications for resuscitation.
   c. Skills in airway management, laryngoscopy, endotracheal intubations, artificial ventilation, suctioning of airways, cardiac massage, biochemical resuscitation, and maintenance of thermal stability. The ability to decompress tension pneumothorax by needle aspirations also is a desirable skill.

4. Procedures should be developed to ensure the readiness of equipment and personnel and to provide for intermittent review and evaluation of the effectiveness of the system.

5. Contingency plans should be established for multiple births and other unusual circumstances.

Apgar Score

At 1-minute and 5-minute intervals after the complete birth of the neonate, Apgar scores (Table 4–1) should be obtained. If the 5-minute score is less than 7, additional scores should be obtained every 5 minutes up to 20 minutes unless two successive scores are 8 or greater.

Table 4–1. Apgar Score

Sign	0	1	2
Heart rate	Absent	Slow (<100/min)	>100/min
Respirations	Absent	Weak cry; hypoventilation	Good, strong cry
Muscle tone	Limp	Some flexion	Active motion
Reflex irritability (response to brisk slap on soles of feet)	No response	Grimace	Cough or sneeze
Color	Blue or pale	Body pink; extremities blue	Completely pink

(Apgar V et al: Evaluation of the newborn infant—Second report. JAMA 168:1985, 1958. Copyright 1958, American Medical Association)

The assignment of the score should be made by a person (e.g., a nurse) not directly involved in resuscitating the neonate. When necessary, resuscitation should be initiated before an Apgar score is obtained. The scores, especially when indicative of a delay in the return of tone, are useful in identifying the neonate who has sustained a significant insult, in assessing the efficacy of resuscitation (change from 1-minute to 5-minute score), and in predicting risks of neonatal and later mortality and morbidity (particularly a low Apgar score at 10, 15, and 20 minutes).

If a low Apgar score is anticipated or detected, rapid assessment of the neonate is necessary in order to define a care plan.

Maintenance of Body Temperature

Immediately following delivery, the neonate should be placed in a warm place and dried completely. Drying the neonate with prewarmed towels immediately after birth reduces evaporative heat loss. A radiant warmer in the resuscitation area is recommended because such devices provide easy access to the neonate during resuscitation procedures.

Suctioning

The mouth may be suctioned gently to remove excess mucus or blood. Vigorous suctioning of the posterior pharynx should be avoided, however, as this might produce significant bradycardia. If there is meconium in the amniotic fluid, the mouth and hypopharynx should be thoroughly suctioned with a DeLee trap or other appropriate device prior to delivery of the shoulders. In the presence of thick or particulate meconium, some authorities feel that the larynx should be visualized and suctioned directly by means of an endotracheal tube; others feel this may be unnecessary, particularly if the mouth and hypopharynx are suctioned thoroughly prior to delivery and if there is no evidence of fetal or neonatal distress. If the neonate is intubated, suction may be applied directly by mouth through a surgical mask to the endotracheal tube and the tube slowly withdrawn (Table 4–2).

Table 4–2. Guidelines for Endotracheal Tubes and Suction Catheters

Weight (kg)	Endotracheal tube (size ID min)	Depth of insertion (cm from upper lip)	Suction catheter size
1	2.5	7	5F
2	3.0	8	6F
3	3.5	9	8F

This procedure may be repeated to ensure removal of as much material as possible.

Resuscitation

The normal neonate breathes within seconds of delivery and has established regular respiration by 1 minute of age. The need for resuscitation is determined by the condition of the neonate. A flaccid neonate who is not breathing spontaneously and whose heart rate is less than 80 beats/minute requires immediate ventilation. A bag and mask can often provide effective ventilation (Fig. 4–2), but this method may be quite difficult to use in premature neonates with noncompliant lungs. If the neonate's heart rate does not rise promptly above 60–80 beats/minute, endotracheal intubation is required. Before applying positive pressure ventilation, it is important to ensure that the airway has been cleared. Initial lung inflation may require 30–40 cm water pressure, but less pressure is needed for succeeding breaths, which should be provided at a rate of 40–60/minute. With rare exceptions, severely asphyxiated neonates respond promptly to adequate ventilation, and this is the only resuscitation maneuver required. Preferably, oxygen should be warmed and humidified.

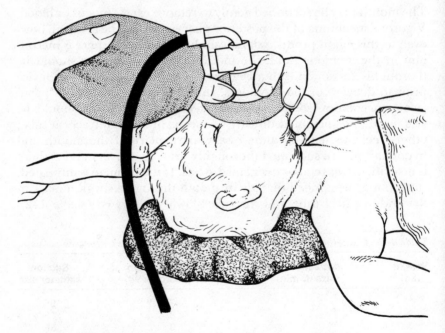

Fig. 4–2. *Artificial ventilation of the newborn with bag and mask.*

Adequacy of ventilation is judged by symmetrical movement of the apices of the chest, equal breath sounds (heard in the axillae), and improvement in heart rate, color, and tone. The response of the heart rate is the most useful and readily measurable criterion of adequate resuscitation. If the response to ventilation is not prompt, the seal between the face and mask or the position of the endotracheal tube should be checked. If chest movement and breath sounds in an intubated neonate appear satisfactory, yet the neonate is not responding, the position of the endotracheal tube should be checked by direct visualization of the larynx with a laryngoscope.

EXTERNAL CARDIAC MASSAGE. If the heart beat does not rise promptly above 60–80 beats/minute following effective ventilation with oxygen, external cardiac massage should be instituted immediately while ventilation is continued. The neonate's chest is encircled with both hands, with the thumbs over the midportion of the sternum (Fig. 4–3). The midportion of the sternum is then compressed ½–¾ in. (1.5–2 cm) at 120 beats/minute. After every third compression, as pressure on the sternum is released, the lungs should be inflated. If there is no response in the heart rate, appropriate drug therapy and volume expansion (if indicated) should be instituted.

DRUGS AND VOLUME EXPANSION. The use of drugs for resuscitation of the neonate is rarely necessary in the delivery room. When they are needed (Table 4–3), they should not be administered until ventilation has been adequately established. The preferred route of administration is the umbilical artery or vein. If a central route cannot be used, intracardiac injections of drugs such as epinephrine might be necessary, but such injections are potentially hazardous.

Acidosis. Severely asphyxiated neonates have a combined metabolic and respiratory acidosis. The treatment of acidosis is treatment of the cause. Thus, respiratory acidosis, which is the result of hypoventilation, is treated by providing positive pressure ventilation. Metabolic acidosis is the result of hypoxemia or hypoperfusion, and the correction of these factors should correct the acidosis. However, significant acidemia is detrimental to myocardial function in the hypoxic heart. If bradycardia or poor perfusion persist in spite of adequate ventilation, 2 mEq/kg sodium bicarbonate may be given. This should be diluted 1:1 with sterile water to a concentration of 0.5 mEq/ml and infused at a rate no greater than 1–2 mEq/kg/minute.

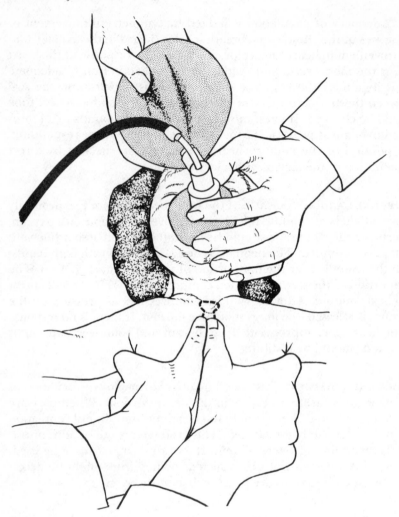

Fig. 4–3. *External cardiac massage.*

Bradycardia. Sodium bicarbonate, epinephrine, calcium gluconate, or atropine may be given (in that order) for bradycardia that persists after adequate ventilation and cardiac massage. Dosages are given in Table 4–3.

Hypovolemia. It is important to recognize that most asphyxiated neonates are not hypovolemic and that there are potential hazards (e.g., intracranial hemorrhage) to overzealous volume expansion. Condi-

Table 4–3. Indications for Drugs in Resuscitation of the Newborn

Indication	Drug	Dose
Metabolis acidosis	Sodium bicarbonate	2 mEq/kg initially
Bradycardia	Epinephrine hydrochloride	0.1 ml/kg of 1:10,000 solution
Low cardiac output	10% calcium gluconate	1 ml/kg
Bradycardia	Atropine sulfate	0.03 mg/kg
Low blood volume	Albumisol	10 ml/kg of 5% solution
Low blood volume	Ringer's lactate	10 ml/kg
Hypoglycemia	Dextrose	2 ml/kg 10%
Respiratory depression secondary to narcotics	Naloxone	0.01 mg/kg

tions associated with hypovolemia include significant hemorrhage from the fetoplacental unit (e.g., vasa previa, fetomaternal bleeding) and compression of the umbilical cord.

Clinical signs of shock might not be apparent until 20%–25% of the blood volume has been lost. If significant hypovolemia is suspected, it should be treated with repeated small infusions of volume expanders (5–10 ml/kg). The neonate's response should be assessed after each infusion. Therapy is stopped when tissue perfusion is adequate. Whole blood (O-negative cross-matched against the mother's blood) is best, but it might not be available. For unanticipated shock, heparinized placental blood may be used; this is obtained from the umbilical cord after it has been sterilized with a solution of 1% tincture of iodine in 70% alcohol. Blood is withdrawn into a 20-ml syringe with 1 ml 50U/ml heparin and administered using a filter from a blood set. Alternatively, 5% albumin or Ringer's lactate may be used.

Narcotic-Induced Respiratory Depression. If respiratory depression is the result of narcotics administered to the mother prior to delivery, naloxone hydrochloride, 0.01 mg/kg, may be administered after assisted ventilation has been and continues to be provided.

NORMAL POSTPARTUM AND NEWBORN CARE

Postpartum hospitalization has several purposes: to identify maternal and neonatal complications, to provide professional assistance during the time when the mother is most likely to be uncomfortable, and to allow adequate time for instruction so the parents may return home with reasonable competence and confidence.

Emphasis in the immediate postpartum period should be placed on the initiation of positive parent-neonate relationships that can be carried over to the home environment. Adequate preparation should include provisions not only for the mother and newborn but also for siblings and other members of the household. This preparation and introduction of other family members can begin in the hospital. To enhance positive interaction with the newborn, liberal visiting privileges for the immediate family are encouraged (see Visiting, this chapter).

Care of the Mother

Immediate Postpartum Care

Postpartum care begins immediately after delivery, in a recovery area or in a birthing room where the woman can be observed for postpartum complications such as hemorrhage or hematoma formation. During this period of observation, maternal blood pressure and pulse should be taken and recorded every 15 minutes for the first hour, and more frequently if the patient's condition warrants. The uterine fundus should be examined frequently to check for excessive bleeding and palpated to determine if it is well contracted. The uterus should be well contracted to minimize bleeding. If the uterus has a tendency to relax or if the patient has a predisposing cause for postpartum hemorrhage (e.g., an overdistended uterus) or a history of postpartum bleeding with a prior pregnancy, a dilute solution of oxytocin should be administered by intravenous drip. If vaginal bleeding occurs or if the patient complains of perineal pain, the cause of the bleeding or pain should be determined by careful palpation of the uterus and by inspection and palpation of the perineum for lacerations or hematoma formation.

The father or other supporting person may remain with the new mother during the immediate postpartum period. Parents should be encouraged to interact with the neonate unless such interaction is precluded by maternal or neonatal complications. When the neonate remains with the mother, an initial assessment of the neonate's condition should be made by the physician or nurse. Routine observations should be initiated and continued during the transitional period to note any conditions, such as respiratory distress or hypothermia, that require special attention.

Following major conduction or general anesthesia for either vaginal or cesarean delivery, the patient should be observed in an appropriately staffed and equipped recovery area until she has recovered from anesthesia. Staff assigned to the recovery area should have no other obligation. The patient should be discharged from the recovery area only at the discretion of the attending physician or the anesthesiologist in charge. A record of vital signs should be maintained and additional signs or events monitored and recorded as they occur.

Subsequent Care

When the patient is taken to her postpartum room, her vital signs, the status of the uterine fundus, and the rate of bleeding should be reassessed and recorded. This assessment should be repeated at regular intervals for the next several hours. The physician should sign the patient's transfer to the postpartum unit after writing the appropriate postpartum orders. While in the postpartum unit, the mother should be taught how to care for herself and her neonate, and problems related to her general health should be discussed. Specific postpartum policies and procedures should be established through cooperative efforts of the medical and nursing staff.

BED REST, AMBULATION, AND DIET. Bed rest is recommended for only a brief time, just long enough to allow the new mother to regain her strength, sleep, and recover from the effects of analgesic or anesthetic agents that she may have received during labor. Intravenous fluids may be required for hydration. Since early ambulation has been shown to decrease the incidence of subsequent thrombophlebitis, the patient should be encouraged to ambulate, with assistance, as soon as she feels able. The patient should not attempt to get out of bed initially without the help of an attendant. A full diet may be given to the mother as soon as she desires it.

CARE OF THE VULVA. The patient should be taught to cleanse the vulva from anterior vulva to perineum and anus rather than in the reverse direction. After repair of episiotomy, initial edema and pain are likely to be reduced during the first 4–6 hours by application of an ice bag. Orally administered analgesics are commonly required and usually are sufficient for relief of discomfort from episiotomy. Pain that is not relieved by such medication suggests hematoma formation and requires a careful examination of the vulva and vagina. Beginning 24 hours after delivery, either dry heat with an infrared lamp or moist heat in the form of a warm sitz bath can be applied to reduce local discomfort and promote healing.

CARE OF THE BLADDER. A woman who has just delivered often has difficulty voiding. This may be related to trauma of the bladder during labor and delivery, regional anesthesia, or pain from the episiotomy site. In addition, the diuresis that may follow delivery may distend the bladder before the patient is aware of the desire to void. To ensure adequate emptying of the bladder, the patient should be checked frequently during the first 24 hours after delivery, with particular attention to displacement of the uterine fundus and any indication of a fluid-filled bladder above the symphysis. Every effort should be made to help the patient void spontaneously; however, a single catheterization may be necessary. An in-dwelling catheter may be preferable to repeated catheterization.

BATHING. After the mother is able to ambulate, she may shower. Tub baths may begin either on the second postpartum day or after discharge from the hospital.

CARE OF THE BREASTS. The mother's decision about nursing her newborn determines the appropriate care of the breasts. Breast care for a woman who chooses to breast-feed is outlined in Chapter 7, Maternal and Newborn Nutrition. The woman who does not desire to breast-feed should be reassured that stopping the milk production is not a major problem. Breast engorgement, which usually occurs in the second or third day following delivery, is not due to milk retention but to accumulation of blood and lymphatic fluid. During the stage of engorgement, the breasts become tense and painful, and they should be supported with a well-fitting brassiere. Ice packs or small doses of analgesics may be required to relieve discomfort during this 12- to 24-hour period. If needed, there are many choices of medication to suppress lactation, most of them hormonal in nature. The benefit/risk ratio of these medications should be detailed to the patient.

TEMPERATURE ELEVATION. The condition of all postpartum patients with an elevated temperature should be evaluated and appropriate cultures taken (see Chapter 6). The nursery should be notified if the mother develops a fever, especially within the first 24 hours, so that the neonate can be evaluated for potential infection.

POSTPARTUM STERILIZATION. Performing tubal ligation immediately after delivery that has been conducted under anesthesia has the advantages of reducing the length of hospitalization and eliminating the need for a second administration of anesthesia. When no anesthesia has been used for delivery, delaying sterilization beyond the first 24 hours does not appear to increase morbidity. If there is an indication of a neonatal problem, the timing of this elective procedure should be reevaluated.

IMMUNIZATION: RhIG AND RUBELLA. An unsensitized Rho(D)-negative woman who delivers an Rho(D)- or D^u-positive neonate is a candidate for prophylaxis and should receive 300 μg RhIG postpartum. The acid elution test for fetal cells in maternal blood to determine the volume of fetal/maternal bleeding should be considered in circumstances such as abruptio placentae and placenta previa, which are known to be associated with a fetal/maternal hemorrhage exceeding 30 ml. If additional RhIG is indicated, it should be administered.

Patients who have received RhIG during the antepartum period (see Laboratory Tests, this chapter) may have a residual passive antibody titer immediately postpartum. This is not a contraindication to standard postpartum prophylaxis in these cases. If the neonate is Rh-positive, a second administration is required, even if the patient has received RhIG during pregnancy.

If a patient has been identified as rubella-susceptible, she should receive the rubella vaccination in the postpartum period. Rubella vaccination can be administered after delivery prior to discharge, even if the patient is breast-feeding.

Care of the Neonate

Most neonates are born after a full-term gestation, are of appropriate birth weight for gestational age, have no congenital defects, and have no illness. However, many neonatal problems manifest themselves during the first 72 hours after birth.

Immediate Stabilization Period

Stabilization usually occurs during the first 12 hours after birth. After appropriate initial care in the resuscitation area, neonates who at birth are sick, small, or at high risk of becoming sick, as determined by history or physical examination, should be transferred to an intermediate or intensive care area.

Following initial evaluation of the neonate's condition, a care plan appropriate to the individual neonate is then established, and the neonate is carefully observed for the next 6–12 hours. Anticipatory observations in the stabilization period include temperature, heart and respiratory rates, blood pressure, color, adequacy of peripheral circulation, type of respiration, level of consciousness, and amount of tone and activity. Observations should be made and recorded at least once per hour until the neonate's condition is stable for 2 hours. Healthy neonates need not leave their mothers for this stabilization period if the facilities used for their observation are in the mother's recovery or postpartum area. Following these careful observations during the first 6–12 hours of life, the neonate who has no identified problem may be placed in the newborn nursery or in the room with the mother for continued observation and care until discharge.

NEONATE IDENTIFICATION. While the newborn is still in the delivery room, two identical bands indicating the mother's admission number, the neonate's sex, and the date and time of birth should be placed on the wrist or ankle. The nurse in charge of the delivery room is responsible for preparing and securely fastening these identification bands to the neonate. The birth records and identification bands should be checked by both the nurse and the responsible physician before the neonate leaves the resuscitation area of the delivery room. When the neonate is admitted to the nursery, both the delivery room nurse and the admitting nurse should check the identification bands and birth records, verify the sex of the neonate, and sign the neonate's record. The admitting nurse should fill out the bassinet card and attach it to the bassinet. Later, when the neonate is shown to the mother, she should be asked to verify the information on the identification bands and the sex of the neonate. It is imperative that delivery room and nursery personnel be meticulous in the preparation and placement of neonate identification bands.

Footprinting and fingerprinting has in the past been recommended for purposes of neonate identification. Techniques such as sophisticated blood typing are now available and appear to be more reliable. If utilized, dermatoglyphics should be done carefully. Individual hospitals may want to continue with footprinting and fingerprinting, but universal use of this practice is no longer recommended.

RISK ASSESSMENT. As soon as possible, and no later than 2 hours after birth, admitting personnel should evaluate the neonate's status and assess risk. Necessary clinical data that were unavailable initially are either obtained or requested at this time. A risk assessment can be determined from the history and physical examination as outlined in the following sections.

History of Maternal Health, Prenatal Course, Labor, and Delivery. The nurse or physician in attendance at delivery should prepare a history, including the following information:

1. History of hereditary conditions in each parent's family
2. Medical history of mother (e.g., diabetes, hypertension, or infection)
3. Past obstetric history (e.g., number, duration, and outcome of previous pregnancies, with dates)
4. First day of the last menstrual period and estimated date of confinement
5. Maternal disease (e.g., diabetes, hypertension, preeclampsia, infections, fever just prior to, at, or following delivery)
6. Mother's blood group and Rh type, with evidence of sensitization or immunization (e.g., administration of RhIG, see Immunization, this chapter)
7. Serologic test for syphilis and cultures for gonorrhea and herpes, including dates performed
8. Drugs taken during pregnancy, labor, and delivery
9. Results of measurements of fetal maturity and well-being (e.g., lung maturity, ultrasonography, intrauterine growth retardation)
10. Duration of ruptured membranes and labor, including length of second stage
11. Method of delivery, including indications for operative or instrumental delivery
12. Placental abnormalities
13. Estimated amount (oligohydramnios, hydramnios) and description (meconium staining; foul-smelling, particulate matter) of amniotic fluid
14. Apgar scores at 1 and 5 minutes, or every 5 minutes until the Apgar score is 7 or above, with particular emphasis regarding the return of tone if it has been altered
15. Description of resuscitation, if required
16. Detailed description of abnormalities and problems occurring from birth until transfer to the admission/observation area

Initial Physical Examination. The admitting nurse or physician should assess the newborn's condition as soon as possible after birth, either in the nursery or in the recovery room. The neonate's physician should examine the apparently normal neonate no later than 12–18 hours after birth and at least every 3 days during the hospital stay. The neonate should be examined within 24 hours of discharge from the hospital. The results of these examinations should be recorded on the neonate's chart and discussed with the parents. This initial examination record should include the following information:

1. Date and time of birth
2. Date, time, and age of neonate at the time of examination
3. Sex
4. Racial origin
5. Birth weight, gestational age, length, and circumference of head
6. Vital signs, including temperature, heart rate, respiratory rate, and blood pressure
7. General appearance, including activity, tone, and cry
8. Skin (e.g., cyanosis, pallor, icterus, rash, plethora, ecchymoses or petechiae, or nonpresenting parts, meconium staining, peeling)
9. Head (size and shape of skull, molding of caput, hematoma, sutures, fontanelle, fracture, evidence of fetal monitoring or blood sampling, and position of jaw)
10. Facies (peculiar or nonpeculiar)
11. Eyes (red reflex, size, shape, placement, firmness, corneal cloudings, cataract, glaucoma)
12. Nose (bridge, patency of nares and choanae)
13. Mouth and pharynx (height, fusion of palate, teeth, short mandible)
14. Neck (length, masses, hairline)
15. Lungs and thorax (respiratory pattern, quality and distribution of breath sounds)
16. Heart (variability of rate, murmur, circulation, capillary refill, and peripheral pulses)
17. Abdomen (scaphoid, distention, abnormal masses, organomegaly)
18. Genitalia (size, ambiguity, descent of testes, pigmentation, meatus, labia, scrotum)
19. Anus (patency, location)
20. Skeletal structure and extremities (clavicles, hips, number of digits, spine, curvature defects, fractures, midline dermal sinus)
21. Neurologic function (posture; type, amount, and symmetry of movement; level of consciousness; reflex symmetry, alteration of tone)

22. Need for isolation (see Chapter 6)

23. Anomalies

Any major or minor anomaly should be recorded. A checklist of significant minor anomalies is shown in Figure 4–4. If three or more minor anomalies on this list are present, major anomalies may be expected in as many as 90% of the newborns.

Birth Weight/Gestational Age Classification. The neonate's gestational age should be calculated from the mother's menstrual history, physical examination, obstetric milestones noted during pregnancy, and the obstetrician's assessment of gestational age (Fig. 4–5). If examination reveals a marked discrepancy in the estimated duration of pregnancy and the physical and neurologic findings, the gestational age should be established on the basis of the physical examination, in conjunction with a composite of relevant obstetric information and observations.

Data from each neonate should be plotted on a birth weight/ gestational age chart. Classification as small, average, or large for gestational age is thus determined. The determination of gestational age and its relationship to weight can be utilized in risk identification for neonatal illness (Fig. 4–6). For example, neonates who are either large or small for gestational age are at relatively increased risk for hypoglycemia and polycythemia, and appropriate tests such as serum glucose screen or hemoglobin are indicated.

Initial and Subsequent Care

The condition of the neonate should be evaluated on admission to the nursery. Initial evaluation includes a review of the neonate's identification, the mother's health prior to pregnancy and during the prenatal and intrapartum periods, the neonate's condition at birth, and the neonate's success in adapting to extrauterine life. Based on this initial assessment, an individualized care plan is then established, and the neonate is carefully observed for the next 6–12 hours until stabilization. Standardized plans are encouraged. Such plans can adequately assure appropriate assessment and care while babies remain with mothers in a recovery or postpartum area.

Healthy neonates born after uncomplicated pregnancies should be assigned to a care plan that includes appropriate observations for the stabilization period and the remainder of the hospital stay. Observations should be made and recorded each 8 hours until discharge, and the specific times of observation should be recorded. Observation for neonatal problems during the first 3 days of life is essential, since approximately one-third of the neonates who require intensive care

1. **Ocular**

_____ epicanthic folds in varying degrees
_____ lateral displacement of inner canthus
_____ downslanting palpebral fissures
_____ true ocular hypertelorism
_____ upslanting palpebral fissures
_____ brushfield spots

2. **Auricular**

_____ cutaneous tags or pits
_____ incomplete helix development
_____ lack of labulus
_____ prominent ears
_____ low-set ears
_____ slanted ears

3. **Hands**

_____ single transverse palmar crease
_____ bridged (modified transverse) palmar crease
_____ short and broad nails
_____ narrow hyperconvex nails
_____ hypoplasia of nail
_____ asymmetry of fingers
_____ short incurred fifth finger (clinodactyly)
_____ camptodactyly (flexion contracture)

4. **Feet**

_____ asymmetry of toes
_____ clinodactyly
_____ short metatarsal with dorsiflexion of hallus (hammer toe)
_____ syndactyly prox. second and third toes
_____ hypoplasia of nails
_____ deep crease between great toe and second toe
_____ wide gap between great toe and second toe

5. **Skin and Hair**

_____ deep dimples or bony promentorils
_____ deep sacral dimple
_____ "punched out" scalp defects
_____ abnormal eyebrows
_____ low hairline
_____ hirsutism (not secondary to failure to thrive)
_____ multiple hair whorls

6. **Miscellaneous**

_____ aberrant frenula of mouth
_____ mild pectus excavatum
_____ short sternum
_____ scrotum extends distally on penis
_____ labile hypoplasia with prominent clitoris

Fig. 4–4. Checklist of significant minor anomalies in the newborn.

	0	1	2	3	4	5
Neuromuscular maturity						
Posture						
Square window (wrist)	90°	60°	45°	30°	0°	
Arm recoil	180°		100°-180°	90°-100°	<90°	
Popliteal angle	180°	160°	130°	110°	90°	<90°
Scarf sign						
Heel to ear						
Physical maturity						
Skin	gelatinous red, transparent	smooth pink, visible veins	superficial peeling &/or rash, few veins	cracking pale area, rare veins	parchment, deep cracking, no vessels	leathery, cracked, wrinkled
Lanugo	none	abundant	thinning	bald areas	mostly bald	
Plantar creases	no crease	faint red marks	anterior transverse crease only	creases ant. 2/3	creases cover entire sole	
Breast	barely percept.	flat areola, no bud	stippled areola, 1-2 mm bud	raised areola, 3-4 mm bud	full areola, 5-10 mm bud	
Ear	pinna flat, stays folded	sl. curved pinna, soft with slow recoil	well-curv. pinna, soft but ready recoil	formed & firm with instant recoil	thick cartilage, ear stiff	
Genitals ♂	scrotom empty no rugae		testes descending, few rugae	testes down, good rugae	testes pendulous, deep rugae	
Genitals ♀	prominent clitoris & labia minora		majora & minora equally prominent	majora large, minora small	clitoris & minora completely covered	

Apgar_____1 min_____5 min
Age at exam _____ (hr)
Race _____ Sex _____
B.D. _____
LMP _____
EDC _____
Gestational age
  by dates _____(wk)
Gestational age
  by exam_____(wk)
Birth weight _____(g)
_____ percentile
Length_____(cm)
_____percentile
Head circum._____(cm)
_____ percentile
Clin. dist._____None_____Mild
_____ Mod._____ Severe

Maturity rating

Score	Weeks
5	26
10	28
15	30
20	32
25	34
30	36
35	38
40	40
45	42
50	44

***Fig. 4–5.** Assessment of neonatal maturity. The assessment is quickly and easily performed because the chart includes measures of physical maturity and measures of passive tone but not active tone. Items are arranged so that a neonate who scored 2 on each item would be 34 weeks. Physical maturity is most accurately assessed in the minutes or hour or so following birth. The score for each item is indicated at the top of the vertical column. However, neuromuscular maturity may be spuriously retarded in the asphyxiated neonate or the neonate obtunded by anesthetic agents or drugs. Thus, neuromuscular maturity rating should be repeated after a day or two. The sum of scores on all the items of physical and neuromuscular maturity provides a maturity in weeks (see lower right). The physical maturity score times 2 provides the neuromuscular maturity in weeks.*

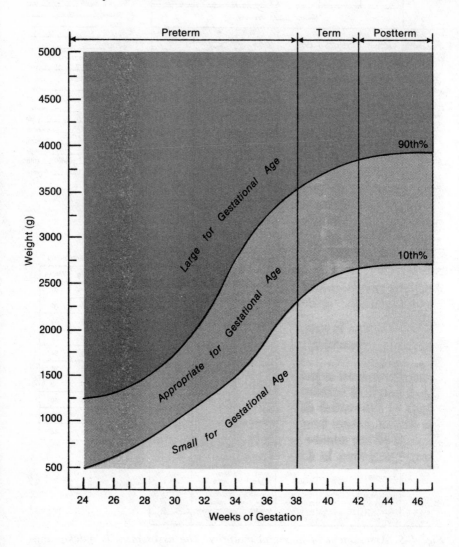

Fig. 4-6. *Birth weight and gestational age for newborns in Colorado. This relation varies with race and altitude. Perinatal units should use the most appropriate data for their location and patient population.*

come from the population of newborns who were free of problems at birth. This 3-day observation period is needed even when the neonate is discharged before 72 hours have elapsed since birth (see Early Discharge, this chapter).

Babies with identified problems or risk factors usually require individualized plans. It is advisable to develop nursery guidelines regarding those conditions (e.g., birth weight, gestational age, or clinical status) that require immediate notification of the physician, direct monitoring activities, or specific actions by nurses before initial physician notification. For example, neonates who are significantly growth-retarded at birth are at risk for hypoglycemia, and their blood glucose levels should be determined periodically. Such determinations can be carried out routinely on growth-retarded newborns admitted to the nursery. Other clinical conditions, such as maternal drug abuse, maternal fever or infection, or low Apgar scores, that are associated with increased risk for neonatal illness, should prompt immediate notification of the physician.

CORD BLOOD. A tube of cord blood should be collected at the time of each neonate's birth. After careful labeling, the blood sample may be refrigerated and stored until the neonate's discharge so that blood type and Rh group can be determined and direct Coombs' or other tests can be done, should they become necessary. Cord blood Rh group should be determined and Coombs antibody tested routinely at the time of delivery if the mother is Rh(D)-negative. Blood typing, Rh determination, and serologic tests for syphilis should be done on cord blood or on blood drawn from the neonate before discharge if the mother was not previously tested.

EYE CARE. One percent silver nitrate in single-dose containers or single-use tubes of sterile ophthalmic ointment containing tetracycline (1%) or erythromycin (0.5%) are acceptable prophylaxes of gonococcal ophthalmia neonatorum. (See Gonococcal and Other Infections in Newborns, Chapter 6.) It should be instilled so it reaches all parts of the conjunctival sac. The eyes should not be irrigated with saline or distilled water after instillation of any of these agents. Instillation may be delayed up to 1 hour following birth (Appendix E).

VITAMIN K. To prevent vitamin K-dependent hemorrhagic disease and coagulation disorders, every neonate should receive a single parenteral dose of 0.5–1.0 mg of natural vitamin K_1 oxide (phytonadione) within 1 hour of birth. There is no advantage to administration of vitamin K to the mother for this purpose.

OBSERVATION. During the remaining stay in the hospital, the neonate should be observed for any sign of illness: (1) temperature instability;

(2) change in activity, including feeding refusal; (3) unusual skin color; (4) abnormal cardiac and respiratory rate and rhythm; or (5) delayed or abnormal voiding and stooling. The normal neonate passes meconium at birth or within the first 24 hours of life. If the neonate has not passed meconium by 48 hours of age, the lower gastrointestinal tract may be obstructed. Urine is normally passed at birth or within the first 12 hours. Failure to void in the first 24 hours may indicate genitourinary obstruction or abnormality, or dehydration.

SKIN AND CORD CARE. This area is of concern mainly because of complications with infections. These considerations are discussed in Chapter 6.

WEIGHING. Each neonate should be weighed at least daily. The neonate must be kept warm during weighing. The scale pan should be covered with a clean paper before each neonate is weighed. The accuracy of the nursery scales should be checked by calibration with a 1-kg weight once a month.

CLOTHING. In addition to a soft diaper, most neonates require only a cotton shirt or gown without buttons. They may be clothed only in a diaper during hot weather if the nursery is not air-conditioned. Cotton blankets used for swaddling should be soft and easily laundered. A supply of clean cotton clothing, bed pads, sheets, and blankets should be kept at the bedside.

Aniline dyes should not be used to mark clothing, blankets, or other items used in the care of newborns.

FEEDING. Under normal circumstances, newborns may nurse as soon as possible after delivery. Breast-feeding is preferred; however, if the neonate is to be fed formula, sterile water is given in the initial reactive period, which is 30 minutes to 2 hours following delivery. All neonates should be given some fluid and nutritional support by at least 6 hours of age. (See Chapter 7 for further details.)

NEONATAL SCREENING. All neonates should be entered into a screening program that meets the following recommendations:

1. An adequate screening program for the persistent hyperphenylalaninemias (PHP), including phenylketonuria (PKU), and for congenital hypothyroidism (CH) in its various forms should ensure (a) total participation by the eligible population, (b) notification of parents about newborn screening and their participation in this

activity, (c) reliable and prompt performance of the screening test, (d) prompt follow-up of subjects with positive tests, (e) accurate diagnosis of subjects with confirmed positive tests, (f) appropriate counseling and treatment of patients.

2. A blood sample should be obtained from every neonate prior to discharge. Siblings of children with PKU/PHP and CH deserve special priority for collection of the sample. An adequate sample is defined as follows: (a) for PKU/PHP, it is heel blood obtained as close as possible to time of discharge from the nursery in a full-term newborn (cord blood is not sufficient); (b) for CH, it is cord blood at birth or heel blood at discharge; (c) in a premature neonate, any neonate receiving parenteral feeding, or any neonate being treated for illness, it is a blood sample obtained at or near the seventh day of age.

3. Neonates initially screened before 24 hours of age should be re-screened for PKU/PHP because cases are more likely to be missed by an initial screening test so soon after delivery. The repeat screening test should be completed before the third week of life.

4. Accurate analysis requires meticulous standardization of the screening method. Accuracy is improved when the cutoff level delineating an abnormal result is defined and specificity of the test is monitored regularly; to do so requires a high volume of samples per unit of time. The analytic component in the program should be centralized to enhance ongoing evaluation of efficiency, accuracy, participation, and adequacy of samples.

5. All patients with PHP should be investigated to rule out the tetra-hydrobiopterin-deficient forms of PKU.

6. Systematic follow-up of neonates with positive CH screening tests is necessary to evaluate the efficacy of CH prevention.

CIRCUMCISION. There is no absolute medical indication for the routine circumcision of the newborn. The procedure of daily stretching of the foreskin is probably not necessary, as many foreskins do not completely retract until the child is 3 years of age. When parents desire the procedure, circumcision should be performed after the first 12–24 hours of the neonatal period. Circumcision should not be performed during the stabilization period after birth.

Parent Education

Parent education is an integral part of the process of childbirth and infant care. The hospital experience is to some extent a learning process, especially for the new mother; hence, it is essential that the physician be willing to accept, understand, and respond to the inquiries of mothers and fathers. Various hospital resources may be helpful to parents, such as closed circuit television films previewed and approved by the obstetric and pediatric staff, printed materials, and counseling by hospital personnel (e.g., postpartum and nursery nurses, registered dieticians/nutritionists, and physical therapists). Group or individual education sessions should be held regularly during the postpartum period to teach and discuss patient self-care, including exercises and self-examination of the breasts; parent-infant relationships; and infant care, including bathing, feeding, and growth and development. Family planning techniques appropriate to the patient's needs and desires should be explained in detail.

The newborn undergoes rapid changes in physiology that should be explained to the parents. The neonate's cardiovascular, pulmonary, renal, and neurologic maturation should be observed by the parents with the guidance of qualified personnel. Parents should be familiar with normal and abnormal changes in wake-sleep patterns, temperature, respiration, voiding, stooling, and the appearance of the skin. They should also observe and become familiar with the behavior, temperament, and neurologic capabilities of the newborn.

Visiting

The father or supporting person may be with the mother as much as desired within the constraints of acceptable standards of care and hospital policy. This includes the labor, delivery (including cesarean delivery), recovery, and postpartum periods. Local policies should be developed and adhered to consistently. Recent trends toward flexibility and liberalization of policies for fathers is encouraged within the context of family-centered care.

Sibling visits may be desirable in the early labor and postpartum periods. Children under 6 years of age frequently experience anxiety when separated from their mother. Contact with the mother and newborn while they are in the hospital helps prepare siblings for a new family member. Physical contact with neonates is a topic of current concern, and no specific recommendations based on data can as yet be made. Through such direct sibling contact, viral infectious diseases may be transmitted to the newborn and, potentially, to other neonates if hospitalization should be prolonged. If siblings are allowed to have direct contact with the newborn, the visit may take place in the mother's private room or in a special sibling visitation area if the mother is not in a private room. Parents should share the responsibility of keeping their newborn from being exposed to a sibling with a contagious illness. Each hospital should develop its own policy regarding sibling visits. Exposure of the newborn to children other than siblings should be avoided.

Other family members and friends should be allowed to visit and see the newborn; however, it may be desirable to restrict such visits to brief periods during the day to avoid disruption of hospital routines. Newborns should be taken to the nursery during this time. Special arrangements may be necessary for other persons important to the new family, such as out-of-town visitors.

Parents of neonates in the continuing care, intermediate care, or intensive care areas should be allowed unrestricted visits whenever possible. Provisions should be made for feeding (particularly breastfeeding), handling, and holding these neonates.

Discharge Planning

The purpose of the postpartum stay is to observe the mother and neonate long enough to identify most maternal and neonatal complications, to provide professional assistance during the time when the mother is most apt to be uncomfortable, and to provide a period of adequate teaching so that the parents may return home with reasonable confidence. Arrangements and specific instructions for postpartum follow-up examinations of both the mother and neonate should be made at the time of discharge. A physical examination and assessment by a physician or physician-associated nurse-practitioner should be scheduled for the neonate on the second or third day of life. (In general, it is preferable for healthy neonates to remain in the hospital more than 24 hours.)

Maternal Considerations

A patient who has had an uncomplicated delivery is usually discharged 48–72 hours after delivery.

The patient should not be discharged until the physician is reasonably certain that there are no major postpartum complications. The patient's vital signs should be stable, and normal bowel and bladder functions should be reestablished. Each patient should be informed of normal postpartum events. The patient should be advised that the normal vaginal discharge from the uterus is termed lochia and that, for the first 2–3 days, it contains a mixture of fresh blood and necrotic debris (lochia rubra). It turns paler (lochia serosa) as bleeding diminishes, and by the seventh day it is yellowish white (lochia alba) because of the predominance of serum and leukocytes. The patient should be informed that the lochia flow diminishes by 3 weeks but may last up to 6 weeks. Anything more than a slight bloody discharge should be reported to the obstetrician. The new mother should be advised on the range of activities reasonable for her to assume; care of the breasts, perineum, and bladder; dietary needs (particularly if she is breast-feeding); exercise; emotional responses; and observations that should be reported to the physician (e.g., temperature elevation, chills, or leg pains).

The time at which coitus may be resumed after delivery is contro-versial. Coitus may cause vaginal laceration and pain if resumed too soon. Risk of hemorrhage and infection are minimal after approxi-mately 2 weeks postpartum; at this time the uterus has involuted markedly, and the endometrium and cervix have begun to reepithel-ize. After 2 weeks postpartum, resumption of coitus may be deter-mined by patient preference and comfort.

If there are no contraindications, oral contraceptive therapy may begin approximately 3 weeks after delivery. Oral contraceptives are contraindicated in the lactating woman until approximately 4–6 weeks after delivery. Neither the intrauterine device nor the diaphragm can be fitted adequately during the immediate postpartum period. Patients who prefer these methods of contraception or patients for whom the use of oral contraceptives is contraindicated should be instructed in the use of methods such as foam and condoms. Methods of contra-ception should then be fully discussed at the 6 weeks' postpartum examination.

Postpartum hospitalization currently averages 2–3 days for nor-mal deliveries. Instructions in the event of a complication or emer-gency should be given at the time of discharge. The roles of the obstetrician, pediatrician, and other members of the health care team concerned with the care of the patient should be delineated clearly. The usual postpartum office visit is made 4–6 weeks after delivery. When there has been a complication during pregnancy or delivery, a 2-week visit is recommended.

Normal Neonates

The family and home must be prepared for the care of the neonate. Mature, healthy newborns are generally discharged at 48–72 hours of age provided the following criteria are met:

1. Transition from intrauterine existence has been successfully com-pleted.

2. The physical examination, performed within at least 24 hours, and preferably within 6 hours of discharge, shows no abnormality.
3. Feeding is adequate with normal stool and urine.
4. Thermal stability has been established.
5. Newborn screening tests have been completed.
6. Methods for obtaining future routine and emergency medical care have been delineated.
7. The home environment is appropriate and those who are to care for the newborn are competent and comfortable.

At the time of discharge, the neonate's condition and instructions for follow-up care should be discussed with the parents. This discussion should include the following points:

1. Condition of the neonate at the time of discharge
2. Immediate needs of the neonate, e.g., feeding methods and environmental supports
3. Future diagnostic and therapeutic plans
4. Future support systems, including psychosocial support systems
5. The physician responsible in case of emergency
6. Reasonable expectations for the future

Early Discharge of Mother and Neonate

Early maternal and neonatal discharge, i.e., within 24 hours of delivery, may be applied on a selective basis. It is preferable that this option be discussed early in the antepartum period. The following criteria should be met:

1. The family and physician should discuss the criteria to be met, and a joint plan by the obstetrician, the pediatrician, and family should be outlined. The agreement should be with the understanding that the course of pregnancy, i.e., antepartum, intrapartum, and early postpartum, will have been uncomplicated and any change in the status of mother, fetus, or neonate during any of these times will alter the plan.
2. The family should have attended prenatal education and neonate care classes that include a discussion of the problems of the first 3–5 days of life.
3. Adequate support systems at home should be identified.

4. The roles of the obstetrician, pediatrician, and other members of the health care team concerned with the continuous medical care of the mother and neonate should be delineated clearly and arrangements made to examine the neonate at 2–3 days of age.

5. The antepartum, intrapartum, and postpartum course for both mother and neonate should be uncomplicated and expected to remain so.

6. The mother should have had a vaginal delivery with no evidence of subsequent hemorrhage or infection. The neonate should be at term (38–42 weeks), normally grown (2500–4500 g), and examined by a physician prior to discharge and found normal.

7. Hospitalization should be a minimum of 6 hours, preferably 12 hours, during which time the neonate has achieved thermal homeostasis and fed successfully (demonstrated normal suck and swallowing mechanisms).

8. Necessary laboratory data should have been obtained, i.e., (a) maternal or cord blood serologic test for syphilis; (b) cord blood (or neonatal blood) type and Coombs' test if the mother is Rh-negative or type O; (c) hemoglobin and blood sugar determinations, if clinically indicated.

9. The mother should demonstrate skill and ability with (a) feeding techniques; (b) skin care, including cord care; (c) temperature assessment and measurement with the thermometer; and (d) assessment of neonatal well-being and recognition of illnesses.

These requirements should be met prior to early discharge. The physician should be aware that the second and ninth criteria may have been met with previous children.

Premature and Sick Neonates

Before discharge, premature and sick newborns not only should meet the criteria listed for mature, healthy newborns, but they also should have

1. Established the ability to maintain adequate fluid and caloric intake independently

2. Shown a satisfactory pattern of growth and development without life support systems

3. Demonstrated thermal stability

4. Had blood drawn for the newborn metabolic screening tests by 7 days of age

A plan for follow-up care should be developed prior to discharge. The physician should be certain that the family has the ability to carry out the plan; in some cases, a training program for the parents is indicated prior to discharge. If the neonate is not to receive follow-up care from the hospital physician, the private physician or agency should be notified that the neonate is to be discharged and should be informed of the recommendations given the parents for the neonate's future care. A written summary should be sent to the neonate's physician.

RESOURCES AND RECOMMENDED READING

Adamsons K Jr: The role of thermal factors in fetal and neonatal life. Pediatr Clin North Am 13:599–619, 1966

American Academy of Pediatrics: Parents—Guidelines for your family's health insurance. Evanston, IL, AAP, 1976

American Academy of Pediatrics, Committee on Drugs: Effect of medication during labor and delivery on infant outcome. Pediatrics 62:402–403, 1978

American Academy of Pediatrics, Committee on Fetus and Newborn: Criteria on Early Infant Discharge and Follow-up Evaluations. Evanston, IL, AAP, 1980

American Academy of Pediatrics, Committee on Genetics: New issues in newborn screening of phenylketonuria and congenital hypothyroidism. Pediatrics 69(1):104–106, 1982

American College of Obstetricians and Gynecologists: Adolescent Perinatal Health: A guidebook for services. Washington, DC, ACOG, 1979

American College of Obstetricians and Gynecologists: Anesthesia for Cesarean Section: Physiologic considerations (ACOG Technical Bulletin 65). Washington, DC, ACOG, 1982

American College of Obstetricians and Gynecologists: Assessment of Maternal Nutrition. Washington, DC, ACOG, 1978, (revised edition, 1982)

American College of Obstetricians and Gynecologists: Care of the Newborn in the Delivery Room (Committee Opinion). Washington, DC, ACOG, 1979

American College of Obstetricians and Gynecologists: Cigarette Smoking and Pregnancy (ACOG Technical Bulletin 53). Washington, DC, ACOG, 1979

American College of Obstetricians and Gynecologists: Diagnostic Ultrasound in Obstetrics and Gynecology (ACOG Technical Bulletin 63). Washington, DC, ACOG, 1981

American College of Obstetricians and Gynecologists: Dystocia: Etiology, diagnosis, and management guidelines (Committee Opinion). Washington, DC, ACOG, 1982

American College of Obstetricians and Gynecologists: Fetal Blood Sampling (ACOG Technical Bulletin 42). Washington, DC, ACOG, 1976

American College of Obstetricians and Gynecologists: Fetal Heart Rate Monitoring: Guidelines for monitoring, terminology and instrumentation (ACOG Technical Bulletin 32). Washington, DC, ACOG, 1975

American College of Obstetricians and Gynecologists: Guidelines on Pregnancy and Work. Washington, DC, ACOG, 1977

American College of Obstetricians and Gynecologists: Guidelines for Vaginal Delivery after a Cesarean Childbirth (Committee Opinion). Washington, DC, ACOG, 1982

American College of Obstetricians and Gynecologists: Immunization During Pregnancy (ACOG Technical Bulletin 64). Washington, DC, ACOG, 1982

American College of Obstetricians and Gynecologists: Induction of Labor (ACOG Technical Bulletin 49). Washington, DC, ACOG, 1978

American College of Obstetricians and Gynecologists: Intrapartum Fetal Monitoring (ACOG Technical Bulletin 44). Washington, DC, ACOG, 1977

American College of Obstetricians and Gynecologists: Obstetric Anesthesia and Analgesia (ACOG Technical Bulletin 57). Washington, DC, ACOG, 1980

American College of Obstetricians and Gynecologists: Precis II: An update in obstetrics & gynecology. Washington, DC, ACOG, 1981

American College of Obstetricians and Gynecologists: Pregnancy, Work and Disability (ACOG Technical Bulletin 58). Washington, DC, ACOG, 1980

American College of Obstetricians and Gynecologists: Prenatal Detection of Neural Tube Defects (ACOG Technical Bulletin 67). Washington, DC, ACOG, 1982

American College of Obstetricians and Gynecologists: Resuscitation of the Newborn. Washington, DC, ACOG, 1977

American College of Obstetricians and Gynecologists: Rubella . . . A Clinical Update (ACOG Technical Bulletin 62). Washington, DC, ACOG, 1981

American College of Obstetricians and Gynecologists: Selective Use of Rho(D) Immune Globulin (RhIG) (ACOG Technical Bulletin 61). Washington, DC, ACOG, 1981

American College of Obstetricians and Gynecologists: Standards for Obstetric-Gynecologic Services, 5 ed. Washington, DC, ACOG, 1982

American Society of Anesthesiologists: Practice Advisory for the Recovery Room. ASA Newsletter 42(5):7–8, May 1978 (ASA Practice Advisory 2).

Amiel-Tison C: Neurological evaluation of the maturity of newborn infants. Arch Dis Child 43:89–93, 1968

Aubrey RH: Identification of the high-risk obstetric patient. In: Ryan GM Jr (ed): Ambulatory Care in Obstetrics and Gynecology. New York, Grune & Stratton, 1980, pp 73–90

Farr V, Mitchell RG, Meligan GA, et al: The definition of some external characteristics used in the assessment of gestational age in the newborn infant. Dev Med Child Neurol 8:507–511, 1966

Hollister Maternal and Newborn Record System. Libertyville, IL, Hollister, 1980

Klaus MH, Fanaroff AA (eds): Care of the High Risk Neonate. Philadelphia, WB Saunders, 1973, p 47

Levine I: Circumcision—Right, rational or both. Patient Care 12(5):72–96, 1978

Levison H, Linsao L, Swyer PR: A comparison of infra-red and convective heating for newborn infants. Lancet 2:1346–1348, 1966

Marx GF, Shnider SM: The obstetric suite. In: American Society of Anesthesiologists: Handbook of Hospital Facilities for the Anesthesiologist, 2 ed. Park Ridge, IL, ASA, 1974, pp 179–184

Mount LE: Radiant and convective heat loss from the new-born pig. J Physiol 173:96–113, 1964

National Foundation–March of Dimes, Committee on Perinatal Health: Toward Improving the Outcome of Pregnancy: Recommendations for the regional development of maternal and perinatal health services. White Plains, NY, National Foundation–March of Dimes, 1977

Nurses Association of the American College of Obstetricians and Gynecologists: Care of the Infant of the Diabetic Mother (Technical Bulletin 11). Washington, DC, NAACOG, 1981

Nurses Association of the American College of Obstetricians and Gynecologists: Guidelines for Childbirth Education. Washington, DC, NAACOG, 1981

Nurses Association of the American College of Obstetricians and Gynecologists: Nursing Histories (Practice Resource). Washington, DC, NAACOG, 1979

Nurses Association of the American College of Obstetricians and Gynecologists: Patient Care Plan: Vaginal delivery, postpartum (Practice Resource). Washington, DC, NAACOG, 1978

Nurses Association of the American College of Obstetricians and Gynecologists: Physical Assessment of the Neonate (Technical Bulletin). Washington, DC, NAACOG, 1978

Nurses Association of the American College of Obstetricians and Gynecologists: Preparation for Parenthood (Technical Bulletin). Washington, DC, NAACOG, 1978

Nurses Association of the American College of Obstetricians and Gynecologists: Standards for Obstetric, Gynecologic, and Neonatal Nursing. Washington, DC, NAACOG, 1981, 2 ed

Nurses Association of the American College of Obstetricians and Gynecologists: A Sample Teaching Guide for the Pregnant Diabetic (Practice Resource). Washington, DC, NAACOG, 1981

Oliver TK Jr: Temperature regulation and heat production in the newborn. Pediatr Clin North Am 12:765–769, 1965

Preston EN: Whither the foreskin? A consideration of routine neonatal circumcision. JAMA 213(11):1853–1858, 1970

Resuscitation of the Newborn (Film). Wheaton, IL, Film and Video Service, 1977

Shnider SM: The anesthesiologist views the design and function of the delivery room. Anesthesiology 37:172–175, 1969

Thompson HC, et al: Report of the Ad Hoc Task Force on Circumcision. Pediatrics 56(4):610–611, 1975

Thompson JE, Clark DA, Salisbury B, et al: Footprinting the newborn infant: Not cost effective. J Pediatr 99(5):797–798, 1981

Usher R, McLean F, Scott KE: Judgment of fetal age: II. Clinical significance of gestational age and an objective method for its assessment. Pediatr Clin North Am 13:835–862, 1966

Wallerstein E: Circumcision: An American health fallacy. New York, Springer, 1980 *chapter*

5
Maternal and Neonatal Follow-Up Care

The postpartum follow-up care of mother and neonate should be coordinated, since procedures and problems that affect one affect the other as well. It should be remembered that the new mother may be unsure of the normal physical changes that occur after delivery and of her ability to care for the newborn. Specific information on postpartum physical changes, the common normal and abnormal newborn states, guidance in newborn care, and appropriate reassurance should be provided prior to discharge. Plans for continuity of care should be developed prior to delivery, reexamined during hospitalization, and rediscussed at the time of the discharge examination. Frequently, a multidisciplinary, collaborative approach is necessary to provide comprehensive health care.

Maternal and neonatal follow-up care should include the following considerations:

1. An assessment of the physical and psychosocial status of both mother and neonate

2. A discussion by the physician or other health professional with the mother (and father, if possible) about expected perinatal problems and ways to cope with them

3. A plan for future care—both immediate and long-range

MATERNAL FOLLOW-UP CARE

Postpartum Evaluation

Postpartum review and examination should be accomplished 4–6 weeks after delivery. This interval should be modified according to the needs of the patient with medical, obstetric, or intercurrent complications.

The first postpartum review should include an interval history and physical examination to evaluate the patient's current status, as well as her adaptation to the newborn. The examination should include an evaluation of weight, blood pressure, breast, abdomen, and the external and internal genitalia. Laboratory data should be obtained as indicated. This is a good time for review of family planning, for determining immunizations, including rubella if not done immediately postpartum, and for discussing any special problems. The patient should be encouraged to return for subsequent periodic examinations.

Psychosocial Adaptive Factors

In the normal postpartum period, the mother's physical and psychic energies move in a predictable course. Initially, the mother's energies are focused on herself and her baby, but they gradually move to encompass others in the immediate environment and eventually extend beyond the immediate surroundings. Care for the new mother during this period should be personalized to hasten the development of a healthy mother-infant relationship and a sense of maternal confidence. Support and reassurance should be provided as the mother masters tasks and adapts to her maternal role. Involving the father and encouraging him to participate in the neonate's care not only provides additional support to the mother but can also enhance the father-infant relationship.

The postpartum period is a time of developmental adjustment for the whole family. Family members now have new roles and relationships, and an effort should be made to assess the progress of the family's adaptation. If a family member—mother, father, or sibling—displays difficulty in assuming the new role, the health care team should arrange for supportive, sensitive assistance.

Supportive Mechanisms and Community Resources

Both in-hospital and community agencies may be needed to assist the developing family. The physician should become familiar with the many public and private groups that give assistance and circumstances under which these organizations might be requested to assist:

1. The in-hospital social service department should be an integral part of the interdisciplinary effort to coordinate hospital and discharge activities, aid in obtaining public or private assistance, and render psychosocial support.

2. Members of the Visiting Nurses Association may be available to visit the home to assess childrearing skills, the home environment,

maternal emotional stability, and infant status and development. Under the physician's direction, these nurses may administer drugs or other therapeutic modalities.

3. Groups that lend support and provide education on special activities, e.g., breast-feeding, are often available.

NORMAL NEONATAL FOLLOW-UP CARE

Information regarding the neonate's condition on discharge should be made available to the physicians who will be providing subsequent care. The newborn should be examined at regular intervals. Weight, length, and head circumference should be measured and plotted on the appropriate graphs to determine normalcy. Blood pressure should be recorded at periodic visits. Efforts should be made to uncover any previously unrecognized congenital anomalies, such as absent femoral pulse, hearing loss, or heart malformations. To identify as early as possible defects that can be ameliorated by intervention, enrichment, or education programs, a neurologic examination should be a part of each visit. Nutritional needs and additions to the diet should be assessed during each visit. Mothers should be informed of normal developmental expectations.

HIGH-RISK NEONATAL FOLLOW-UP CARE

In addition to the usual medical and psychosocial surveillance required for normal neonates, those at risk require a systematic, detailed examination to identify possible physical or psychological disability. As discussed in Chapter 1, follow-up programs are an intergral part of regional perinatal care systems; they provide a base for outcome evaluation and research.

The following perinatal conditions are among those that may identify a significant number of infants at risk:

1. Weight less than 1500 g at birth or gestation less than 34 weeks
2. Small-for-gestational-age status
3. Perinatal asphyxia
4. Apgar score less than 3 at 5 minutes with clinical evidence of neurologic dysfunction
5. Delay in onset (or loss) of spontaneous respiration for more than 5 minutes requiring mechanical ventilation
6. Clinical evidence of central nervous system abnormalities, i.e., seizures, hypotonia, or intraventricular hemorrhage

7. Hyperbilirubinemia of greater than 20 mg/dl in nonsick term neonates (the level of hyperbilirubinemia that causes deficits in premature neonates is unknown). (See Chapter 10)
8. Specific genetic, dysmorphic, or metabolic disorders or a history of such disorders in the infant, a sibling, or other relative
9. History of prenatal or newborn infection
10. Psychosocial abnormalities, e.g., infants of drug-addicted or alcoholic mothers

Care of the infant with documented problems during the perinatal period should include special attention to the nervous system, visual and hearing assessments, sequential development, social behavioral assessment, and the need for early intervention. In the preterm infant, the immunization schedule recommended by the American Academy of Pediatrics should be implemented on an individual basis, considering the infant's general state of health, growth, and development. The time of immunization may be as early as 8 weeks from birth (see Immunization of Premature Infants, Chapter 6).

Neurologic Evaluation

The focus of the neurologic examination changes with age and can be separated into two distinct time periods:

1. Age 0–12 months
   a. Major motor deficits
   b. Seizure disorders
   c. Deafness
   d. Retrolental fibroplasia
   e. Head growth abnormalities
   f. Congenital anomalies, e.g., congenital eye defects such as glaucoma and cataracts
2. Age 1–5 years
   a. Fine and gross motor deficiencies, including balance difficulties
   b. Visual perceptual deficiencies
   c. Myopia, hyperopia, and strabismus
   d. Mild hearing loss
   e. Language difficulties, receptive or expressive
   f. Behavioral problems, e.g., hyperkinesis, high anxiety level, or short attention span

Utilization of a diagnostic assessment timetable (Table 5–1) should

Table 5.1. Diagnostic Assessment Timetable

Age of evaluation	Metabolic screening test	Physical growth	Neurologic assessment	Ophthalmologic assessment	Auditory assessment	Bayley motor mental[†]	Behavioral questions	Zimmerman[‡]	Beery visual motor Integration[§]	Stanford—Binet,[¶] McCarthy,[#] Murphy—Durrell, WISC[**]
Birth	+	+	+							
6 mo*		+	+	+	+	+ +	+			
12 mo*		+	+	+	+	+ +	+			
2 yr*		+ +	+ +			+ +	+ +			
3 yr		+	+				+			
4 yr		+	+				+	+	+	+
5 yr		+	+				+	+	+	‡‡

*Corrected age
[†]Bayley N: Bayley Scale of Infant Development. New York, The Psychological Corp, 1969
[‡]Zimmerman JH: Preschool Language Scale. Columbus, OH, Charles E. Merrill, 1969
[§]Beery KE: Developmental Test of Visual Motor Integration. Chicago, Follett Educational Corp, 1967
[¶]Terman LM, Merrill MA: Stanford–Binet Intelligence Scale. Boston, Houghton–Mifflin, 1973
[#]McCarthy M: McCarthy Scales of Children's Abilities. New York, The Psychological Corp, 1972
[**]Wechsler Intelligence Scale for Children
[‡]Choice of Stanford Binet, McCarthy, or Wechsler
[‡‡]Murphy–Durrell reading readiness analysis (optional)

ensure the identification of major abnormalities by 12 months of age and less serious abnormalities during the subsequent visits. Physicians should not only evaluate the infant's condition, but also be aware of and sensitive to the parents' feelings.

Visual Assessment

See Clinical Considerations in the use of Oxygen, Chapter 10.

Hearing Assessment

Infants with any of the following characteristics are considered at risk for hearing loss:

1. Family history of childhood hearing impairment
2. Congenital perinatal infection (e.g., cytomegalovirus, rubella, herpes, toxoplasmosis, syphilis)
3. Anatomic malformations involving the head or neck, (e.g., dysmorphic appearance including syndromal and nonsyndromal abnormalities, overt or submucous cleft palate, and morphologic abnormalities of the pinna)
4. Birth weight less than 1500 g
5. Hyperbilirubinemia at a level exceeding indications for exchange transfusion
6. Bacterial meningitis, especially that caused by *Hemophilus influenzae*
7. Severe asphyxia, which may be exhibited by neonates who have Apgar scores of 0–3 or who fail to institute spontaneous respiration by 10 minutes of age, as well as by those with hypotonia persisting for 2 hours of age

The hearing of infants who manifest any characteristic item on the list of risk criteria should be screened, preferably under the supervision of an audiologist, and optimally by 3 months of age but no later than 6 months of age. The initial screening should include the observation of behavioral or electrophysiologic response to sound. If consistent responses are detected at appropriate sound levels, the screening process is considered complete, except when there is a probability of a progressive hearing loss, e.g., a family history of delayed onset or degenerative disease, or a history of intrauterine infection. If results of an initial screening are equivocal, the infant should be referred for diagnostic testing.

Diagnostic hearing evaluation of an infant less than 6 months of age should include a general physical examination and history encompassing the following evaluations:

1. Examination of the head and neck
2. Otoscopy
3. Identification of relevant physical abnormalities
4. Laboratory test, such as urinalysis and diagnostic tests for perinatal infections

Comprehensive audiologic evaluation should include (1) a behavioral history, (2) behavioral observation audiometry, and (3) testing of auditory evoked potentials, if indicated.

After the age of 6 months, communication skills evaluation, acoustic impedance measurements, and selected tests of development are also recommended.

Hearing and speech and language function should be screened periodically. Hearing may be roughly evaluated by the startle response during the newborn period. At 6–9 weeks, an infant should turn the head toward a familiar sound. At 12 months, a child should understand simple directions and a few words such as "Mama," "no," or "hot." A comprehensive auditory evaluation should be obtained if the infant's responses are inadequate.

Developmental Assessment

Specific developmental tests are used to assess gross motor, fine motor, language, and personal social adaptive behavior from birth to 5 years. The Denver Developmental Screening Test, for example, provides a simple method of screening for developmental delays. This test is designed to alert professionals to the need for an in-depth evaluation if development is shown to be deficient in any area. The Bayley Scale of Infant Development is probably the most standardized test available for infants between 6 months and 2 years of age. At 3 years, both the Stanford-Binet Intelligence and the McCarthy Cognitive Index are acceptable standardized tests that can be used to assess cognitive functioning, although physical handicaps may invalidate the test. At age 4 years or older, some psychologists find the Beery Visual Motor Integration (VMI) and Zimmerman Receptive Expressive Language Assessment useful in identifying specific problems that require early education programs.

Social Behavioral Assessment

A problem-oriented questionnaire on the family background may alert the physician to nonmedical risk factors that ultimately may affect family stability and the adequacy of child care. Such a questionnaire should include the following information:

1. Developmental stage of the parents, e.g., teenage, young adult, or adult
2. Level of education of parents
3. Parental attitude and behavior
4. Changes in parent-child interaction since last visit
5. Sibling problems
6. Major stresses or changes in lifestyle
7. Spouse relationship
8. Problems with other agencies
9. Problems with "significant" people
10. Income
11. Other responsible adults
12. Areas where help is needed

Social-behavioral questions relevant to the at-risk family and infant may be used to assess the presence of (1) behavior that is normal, (2) behavior that causes family disruption, and (3) behavior that is developmentally incapacitating. Prolonged hospitalization inevitably disrupts the family and has been demonstrated to have an effect on the parent-child relationship. Information on social status and familial characteristics is also important because these factors are known to affect psychomotor performance, especially language development. Identification of family relationships at risk is important because it permits intervention and referrals for counseling, mental health services, and parent support groups.

Early Intervention and Education

In recent years, it has been postulated that early identification, intervention, support, stimulation, training, and education may improve the social adaptation of handicapped infants and their families. A follow-up program offers a unique opportunity to screen an at-risk population and make appropriate referrals of infants with specific neurodevelopmental or neurosensory handicaps to intervention or therapeutic programs. The effectiveness of early intervention programs is being studied.

CHILD ABUSE

Physicians and other health care workers who provide follow-up care to mothers and infants should be aware that there are physical and psychosocial factors that are associated with an increase in child abuse. The following factors are part of an evolving list that should continually be evaluated:

1. Prematurity
2. Illness with long periods of hospitalization in the neonatal intensive care unit
3. Single parents, particularly the adolescent mother
4. Infrequent visitation by families of hospitalized infants

Closer follow-up of these infants and their parents is required. The interaction of the parents, particularly the mother, with the infant should be evaluated. Health personnel in perinatal units should be aware of contributing factors and be knowledgeable and sensitive to normal and abnormal reactions of the mother to her infant.

RESOURCES AND RECOMMENDED READING

American Academy of Pediatrics: Report of the Committee on Infectious Diseases, 19 ed. Evanston, IL, American Academy of Pediatrics, 1982

Joint Committee on Infant Hearing: Position statement 1982. Pediatrics 70(3):496–497, 1982

6

Control of Infections in Obstetric and Nursery Areas

Infections may affect either mother or neonate or both during the perinatal period. They are relatively uncommon in healthy mothers who deliver vaginally at term or in normal newborns, however. Women who have had a complicated pregnancy and labor or a cesarean delivery are much more likely to develop infection, and sick or preterm neonates in the intensive care unit may have high rates of nosocomial infection. In some intensive care nurseries, 15% or more of the neonates may have one or more infections; a high percentage of these infections may be fatal.

Most infections in obstetric patients are caused by endogenous flora—microorganisms that are normally resident in the genital tract but generally cause invasive disease only during labor, delivery, or the puerperium. Many of these infections can be prevented through meticulous surgical and patient care techniques and appropriate use of prophylactic antibiotics. Bacterial pathogens such as group B streptococci or *Listeria monocytogenes,* if acquired by neonates from their mothers during birth, occasionally cause pneumonia or septicemia during the first hours or days of postnatal life. At present, these infections are difficult to predict or prevent, although they occur more frequently after prolonged rupture of membranes or a complicated labor and delivery. In contrast, most infections in neonates in intensive care units are caused by pathogens acquired from the hospital environment. Prevention of these infections requires a multifaceted approach, including careful attention to patient care techniques, elimination of inappropriate antibiotic use to avoid further alteration of the balance of colonizing flora, and careful attention to all aspects of infection control.

COLONIZATION OF NEWBORN INFANTS

Most neonates are born from a sterile intrauterine environment; during and after birth, they are exposed to the first of numerous microorganisms that will colonize their skin, nasopharynx, gastrointestinal tract, and other areas. Many factors, some of which can be modified by medical personnel and hospital procedures, influence the types of colonizing organisms, the balance of the organisms, and the host response to the organisms.

Ill neonates who are subjected to multiple invasive procedures in an intensive care unit are frequently colonized at multiple sites with a variety of organisms, particularly gram-negative bacteria. Full-term, healthy neonates who are handled almost exclusively by their mothers are unlikely to have severe infections. The exceptions to this are that infections secondary to group B streptococci, *Escherichia coli* (K1 antigen), *L. monocytogenes, Salmonella, Chlamydia,* herpes simplex virus, or enteroviruses may be severe. These organisms subsequently may be transmitted to other neonates in the nursery on the hands of hospital personnel.

The bowel flora of a neonate who is breast-fed exclusively is qualitatively and quantitatively different from that of a neonate who is formula-fed, especially if the latter is fed via continuous drip feedings administered by hospital personnel.

The skin of the newborn is a major initial site of bacterial colonization, particularly with *Staphylococcus aureus;* colonizing strains of this organism are most commonly transmitted within the nursery rather than from the mother. Any break in the integrity of the protective skin affords an opportunity for infection to develop. At birth, for example, a neonate has at least one open surgical wound (the umbilicus) that is highly susceptible to infection. A circumcision site is another area that could become infected.

The importance of bacterial interference in preventing infection in the newborn has not yet been fully explored, and future investigations in this area may change not only medical practice but also the risk of infection in the newborn.

Since many organisms may be pathogenic for the neonate, nursery personnel need to recognize the importance of patient care techniques in limiting the spread of organisms from one neonate to another within the nursery. It is not necessary to restrict nursery admissions to infants born under "sterile" conditions. Those born under "unsterile" conditions (or after prolonged rupture of membranes or to mothers with suspected or proved infection), those transferred from another hospital, or those readmitted after discharge may be admitted to most nurseries if precautions are taken to prevent transmission of colonizing or infecting organisms from one neonate to another. Similarly, neonates may be moved safely from one nursery area to another under normal circumstances. Arbitrarily categorizing neonates as "clean" or "dirty," based on their experiences during delivery or the presence of confirmed infection, may lead to the assumption that the "clean" neonates do not harbor organisms that can cause disease, and this may result in inappropriate care. It is important, however, to approach the care of each neonate as if he or she were colonized with unique flora that should not be transmitted to any other neonate and to protect each neonate from the flora of all others.

Neonates who require intensive care undergo a variety of invasive procedures—intubation with ventilation or other respiratory tract care, intravascular lines, nasogastric or nasoduodenal tubes—that breach normal barriers to infection and provide additional opportunities for colonization. Depending on circumstances, most neonates colonized with pathogenic organisms do not have overt signs of illness and are not managed with special precautions. Those neonates in the same nursery who have not yet been colonized are highly susceptible to colonization and infection and frequently acquire their organisms as physicians, nurses, respiratory therapy personnel, and other personnel move from one neonate to another. Because of this, a high proportion of the neonates in a single nursery may be colonized or infected with the same strain; respiratory tract and intestinal organisms are particularly common in such situations. To minimize transmission of organisms, each individual working with these neonates and with the equipment used directly in their care should be meticulous when providing patient care. After taking care of a neonate, personnel should wash their hands before taking care of another neonate or the same neonate at another site, and they should dispose of contaminated equipment or materials properly.

SURVEILLANCE FOR NOSOCOMIAL INFECTION

The infection control committee of each hospital should work with the perinatal personnel to establish workable definitions of nosocomial infection for surveillance purposes. For obstetric patients, a nosocomial infection can be broadly defined as one that is neither present nor incubating at the time the patient is admitted to the hospital. Most cases of endometritis or urinary tract infection that occur postpartum, therefore, are nosocomial, even though the causative organisms may be endogenous.

Nosocomial infection in newborns is more difficult to define. The broadest definition includes all infections that have an onset after birth, excluding only those known to have been transmitted transplacentally. Narrower definitions exclude those infections that develop within 24–72 hours of birth, since these too may have been caused by organisms acquired from the mother rather than from the hospital environment. The narrower, more specific definitions are probably more useful for general purposes. Definitions should include neonates with onset of disease during a period after discharge. The definition selected should be applied consistently to allow uniform reporting and analysis of nosocomial infections.

Obstetric and nursery personnel should cooperate with the hospital infection control personnel in conducting and reviewing the results of surveillance programs for nosocomial infections. This type of monitoring provides information about the occurrence of unusual problems or clusters of infection, the risks involved with certain procedures or techniques, and the success of specific preventive measures. Generally, the surveillance program can be conducted most efficiently if it emphasizes detection of infections in hospitalized patients, although most postpartum women and their newborns are discharged after only a few days in the hospital. Routine culturing of neonates for surveillance purposes is not recommended, but cultures of lesions or sites of infection can be helpful in identifying clusters of infection caused by a single strain of bacteria. Since infections with organisms acquired within the nursery may not become apparent until after discharge of the newborns, it is especially important for pediatricians and others caring for newborns to report confirmed or suspected postdischarge infections to nursery and hospital infection control personnel.

Patterns of infections are easier to identify if only those infections involving a specific site or pathogen are included in the data. Usually, only clinically apparent infections should be recorded in the surveillance data; at times, especially during an outbreak, it may be important to detect colonization of all neonates at certain sites or with certain organisms. Distinguishing between colonization and disease at a site such as the lower respiratory tract is frequently difficult in neonates. Clusters of infection that do not fit a standard definition may need to be individually investigated.

Both obstetric and nursery personnel are involved in providing perinatal care; therefore, good communication between these groups about infectious diseases or other problems is essential. In particular, nursery personnel should be notified in advance about the birth of a neonate with a possible congenital or perinatal infection, and obstetric personnel should be informed about problems in newborns that may be associated with labor and delivery.

MEASURES FOR PREVENTION AND CONTROL OF INFECTIONS

Health Standards for Personnel

Obstetric and nursery personnel, as well as others who have significant contact with the newborn, should be free of transmissible infectious diseases. Each hospital should establish policies and procedures for assessing the health of personnel, restricting contact of personnel with patients when necessary, maintaining employee health records, and reporting illness in personnel. Personnel assigned to the perinatal services should have at least an annual health assessment, including a screening test for tuberculosis. Routine culturing of personnel is not useful, although selective culturing may be of value in special situations.

Personnel should be aware that even a mild transmissible infection may preclude contact with neonates. In general, individuals with a respiratory, cutaneous, mucocutaneous, hepatic, gastrointestinal, or other communicable infection should not have direct contact with neonates.

The risk posed by nursery and other perinatal personnel who have active herpes simplex virus (HSV) infections, such as cold sores, is unknown. HSV has been isolated from the saliva of many asymptomatic personnel, but it is not known whether these individuals pose a greater or lesser risk of infection to neonates than those with clinically apparent infection. Individuals with labial herpes should not kiss or nuzzle neonates. Those with herpetic hand infections (herpetic whitlow) should not provide direct patient care, particularly for neonates, until the lesions have healed. Personnel with genital HSV infections probably pose little or no risk to patients. In general, the risk of compromising patient care by excluding personnel who are essential for the operation of the unit should be weighed against the potential risk of infecting neonates.

Personnel in contact with neonates should report personal infections or symptoms to their immediate supervisors and be medically examined before working directly with neonates. Dispositions must be individualized; exclusion from obstetric and nursery areas is appropriate for highly contagious conditions, even if the individual feels well enough to continue working. Employee health policies should be arranged so that personnel feel free to report infectious problems without fear of income loss.

All employees susceptible to rubella should be vaccinated. This may involve a significant proportion of hospital and medical personnel, both men and women. Those working in the obstetric and nursery areas, including clinics, may be exposed to persons or neonates with rubella infection or may themselves transmit infection to pregnant women. To protect the fetuses of pregnant employees, susceptible women in the childbearing age group must be identified and offered vaccine before they become pregnant or are exposed to infected infants. Vaccine should not be administered to pregnant women; conception should be avoided for 3 months after vaccination.

Personnel in neonatal units are likely to be exposed to patients who are excreting cytomegalovirus; whether these staff members have a greater risk of acquiring primary cytomegalovirus infection is unknown. Since the majority of cytomegalovirus infections are subclinical, previous infection and the current immune status of the exposed person are usually unknown. Women of childbearing age who work in neonatal units should be counseled about the relative risks of exposure should they become pregnant. These women may be offered the opportunity to work in other areas of the hospital during pregnancy. A routine program of serologic testing for obstetric or nursery hospital employees cannot be recommended, although serologic testing may indicate whether an individual has had a prior infection; a rise in antibody titer indicates recent cytomegalovirus infection.

It is desirable to recruit and maintain a regular group of nurses with specialized training in obstetric and nursery nursing to work in these specialty areas. If nurses from other areas must work in the obstetric and nursery areas, or if nurses from the obstetric and nursery areas work on other units of the hospital, specific policies should be established for this practice. Nursing personnel should be assigned for an entire shift and should not be moved back and forth indiscriminately. Nursing personnel from obstetrics and the nursery who work on other units should be assigned to work only with uninfected patients.

Hand-Washing

As mentioned earlier, most of the common infectious agents responsible for colonization and disease in patients, especially in the nursery, are transmitted from patient to patient on the hands of personnel. Therefore, to minimize this type of transmission, medical and hospital personnel must be meticulous about hand-washing.

Before handling neonates for the first time on a shift, personnel should wash hands and arms to above the elbow with an antiseptic agent. Hands should be rewashed before and after handling each neonate and after touching objects or surfaces likely to be contaminated with virulent microorganisms or hospital pathogens (including the hair, face, and clothing of personnel; diapers; and equipment). Routine, brief activities for the care of adult patients may not require hand-washing before each contact. Hands should be washed with the proper technique and with an appropriate agent. Hand-washing materials and facilities must be easily accessible. (See Scrub Areas, Chapter 2.)

Agents for Hand-Washing

Antiseptic (antimicrobial) hand-washing agents have traditionally been recommended for personnel who care for neonates. Antiseptic preparations should be used for scrubbing before entering the nursery, before providing care for neonates highly susceptible to infection, before performing invasive procedures, and after providing care for infected neonates. These preparations may not be essential, however, for routine hand-washing within the nursery; soap and water may be sufficient.

The ideal antiseptic agent for hand-washing should kill pathogenic bacteria; be nonstaining, nonirritating to the skin, and nonsensitizing; and have persistent local action. It should also be easy to use. These requirements limit the number of useful preparations.

The antiseptics most useful for hand-washing in the nursery are chlorhexidine gluconate or iodophor (water-soluble complexes of iodine with surfactant agents) preparations; both are useful against gram-negative and gram-positive organisms. Hexachlorophene-based preparations may be especially useful during nursery outbreaks of *S. aureus* infection. All of the antiseptic compounds are occasionally sensitizing or irritating, and some personnel may need to use plain soap or mild detergents. Liquid soap dispensers and many hand-washing agents may become contaminated; disposable brushes or pads that contain an antiseptic hand-washing agent avoid this problem.

Alcohol-containing foams are satisfactory for degerming the skin; they may be satisfactory when applied to clean hands, but they are not sufficient for cleaning physically soiled hands.

Techniques of Hand-Washing

For the initial 2-minute wash before handling neonates, sleeves should be rolled above the elbows. A small amount of antiseptic preparation should be placed in the palm of the hand, and the hands, wrists, forearms, and elbows washed thoroughly; all areas should be covered, including between fingers and the lateral surfaces of the fifth fingers. Following this initial wash, the fingernails should be cleaned with a plastic or orangewood stick, and the hands washed again (a soft brush or firm pad are optional but not required). After the hands have been washed, they should be rinsed thoroughly and dried with paper towels.

A 15-second wash, without a brush but with soap and vigorous rubbing, is required between handling of neonates or after touching contaminated articles or surfaces. This type of wash usually eliminates most organisms transiently colonizing the hands, although it may not be adequate if the hands are heavily contaminated.

Dress Codes

Each hospital should establish dress codes for regular and part-time personnel entering the labor, delivery, and nursery areas of the hospital. The following recommendations are offered.

Scrub Suits or Dresses

Physicians, nursing personnel, and others who spend most of their working day in the labor, delivery, or nursery areas preferably should wear short-sleeved scrub gowns or short-sleeved scrub suits or dresses provided and laundered by the hospital. The examiner's clothing or unscrubbed portions of the body should not contact neonate or equipment. Fathers attending births also should be in scrub clothes.

Caps and Masks

Although caps, beard bags, and masks are not needed for routine activities in the labor and nursery areas, they are required for delivery and may be beneficial for surgical procedures performed in the nursery, including umbilical vessel catheterization. Long hair must be restrained so that it does not touch the neonate or equipment during patient examination or treatments. Personnel who touch their hair, beard, mustache, or face while on duty should rewash their hands before touching a patient or the patient's equipment.

Masks for personnel are not usually essential to prevent acquisition or dissemination of respiratory pathogens. Masks have limitations.

High-efficiency disposable masks should be used, but even these masks remain efficient for only a few hours. Masks should cover both the nose and the mouth. They should be either completely on or completely off; they should be discarded as soon as they are removed from the nose and mouth. Masks may not be effective on persons who have beards.

Gowns

Sterile, long-sleeved gowns should be worn by all personnel who have direct contact with the sterile field during vaginal deliveries, surgical obstetric procedures, and surgical procedures in the nursery.

In many nurseries where neonates are cared for in bassinets or open beds, visitors or physicians, nursing personnel, and technicians not regularly assigned to the nursery are required to wear short-sleeved gowns to cover their clothing; the need for this type of gowning as a routine infection control measure is not confirmed, however. In nurseries where all neonates are kept in forced-air, isolation-type incubators, personnel who work intermittently in the nursery need not wear gowns.

If an infected or potentially infected neonate is to be handled outside the bassinet, a long-sleeved gown should be worn over the scrub suit or dress, gown, or other clothing and either discarded after use or maintained for exclusive use in the care of a single neonate. If one gown is used for each neonate, the gown should be changed every 8 hours.

When leaving the obstetric or nursery area for other hospital areas (e.g., laboratories, radiology department, or cafeteria), personnel in scrub suit or dress should wear a long-sleeved gown that is discarded on reentering the obstetric or nursery area.

Gloves

Sterile gloves should be used during deliveries and all surgical procedures in either the obstetric or nursery area.

Disposable, nonsterile gloves may be useful in the care of patients in isolation or during other procedures that may result in heavy contamination of the hands. Use of gloves in such circumstances may reduce the intensity of transient bacterial or viral colonization of the hands of patient care personnel.

Jewelry

Personnel should remove rings, watches, and bracelets before washing their hands and entering the obstetric or nursery area; they should not wear jewelry while on duty.

Preventive Measures on an Obstetric Service

In the past few years, many hospitals have relaxed their requirements regarding attire and conduct in the labor area. Since most infections arise from the patient's genital tract flora, this relaxation of regulations is reasonable. Infection control practices such as hand-washing and changing contaminated scrub suits should not be ignored, however. Fathers have also been permitted in the labor and delivery area without any increase in the rates of infections, although the delivery area must be considered a sterile area, especially when cesarean deliveries and tubal ligations are done in the same rooms as vaginal deliveries are done.

Family-centered perinatal programs and use of in-hospital birthing rooms are not associated per se with a higher risk of infection in either mother or neonate.

Surgical Technique

A primary principle in preventing postoperative infection is good surgical technique. Before surgery, the operative field should be prepared and draped. Shaving, when necessary, should be done no earlier than 2 hours before surgery.

Vaginal Examinations

Vaginal examination during labor is not associated with a higher infection rate than is rectal examination; however, the greater the number of examinations, the greater risk of maternal infection.

Preparation for Obstetric Emergencies

Surgical packs, solutions, and other materials and supplies can be kept sealed but conveniently arranged so that the instrument table can be ready almost immediately for an obstetric emergency. Some hospitals keep a surgical pack and tray open and covered with a sterile drape, ready at all times for an emergency cesarean delivery; no studies have established the probability of contamination of the instrument table nor the frequency with which the instruments and equipment should be replaced. In the absence of data on which to base a different recommendation, the instruments and equipment should be replaced at the beginning of each nursing shift.

Intrauterine Pressure and Fetal Monitoring

Intrauterine monitoring requires rupture of the amniotic membranes. Because of the attendant risk of infection in either the mother or the newborn, the catheter and leads should be carefully inserted by means of aseptic technique. Sterile equipment should be used for all fluid pathways in the pressure-monitoring system; the system should be closed, and extreme caution should be used to avoid contamination during procedures such as calibration.

Transducers for intravascular or intrauterine pressure monitoring have caused nosocomial infections for a variety of reasons. Contamination of equipment and subsequent infections in patients have resulted from inadequate cleaning and sterilization of reusable equipment, from the reuse of disposable transducer domes, and from suboptimal techniques as the equipment was assembled and used. To minimize the chance of inadvertent contamination of fluids and equipment, the components of the monitoring system should not be removed from sterile packages and set up until the system is actually needed. After use, all disposable equipment should be discarded and the transducer disinfected (if used with a disposable dome that isolates the head of the transducer from the fluid path) or cleaned and sterilized (if a reusable dome-transducer combination is used).

The application of fetal scalp electrodes inserted through the birth canal of a woman with clinical or subclinical genital HSV infection may transmit HSV infection directly to the fetus.

Prophylactic Antibiotics for Obstetric Patients

Prophylactic antibiotics decrease the frequency of infections in selected high-risk patients. For cesarean delivery in patients with a high risk of infection, short courses of prophylactic antibiotics significantly decrease the incidence of operative site infections and may also decrease the length of hospital stay. Various antibiotic regimens have been effective; a 1-day or 3-dose course is as effective as a longer course. Beginning antibiotic therapy after clamping the cord has been as effective as beginning it before surgery.

A number of objections remain to routine antibiotic prophylaxis during cesarean delivery. First, if infection occurs after prophylaxis, organisms may be more resistant. Second, antibiotics administered intrapartum or before the cord is clamped may alter results of blood cultures or delay diagnosis of infection in the newborn. Third, it is not clear whether prophylactic antibiotics for cesarean delivery prevent a high proportion of serious infections.

It is currently recommended that antibiotic prophylaxis be reserved for patients who must undergo a surgical procedure and who are at a high risk of infection or for patients in whom the consequences of infection would be life-threatening. Antibiotics are not indicated for routine use in most elective cesarean deliveries. In addition, prophylactic antibiotics should be continued for no longer than 24 hours after surgery. The antibiotic chosen for prophylaxis should have a reasonable spectrum of activity against pelvic flora and should be relatively nontoxic. Finally, important therapeutic antibiotics, such as penicillin, aminoglycosides, and clindamycin, should not be used for prophylaxis.

Special Preventive Techniques and Procedures for Neonates

Invasive Procedures on Neonates

Providing care for a sick newborn demands the use of multiple invasive techniques for diagnosis, monitoring, and therapy. Frequently used procedures include assisted ventilation, total parenteral nutrition through a central venous line, umbilical or other arterial cannulation to monitor intravascular pressure and obtain arterial blood gas specimens, and continuous gastric and transpyloric feedings (see Feeding Low-Birth-Weight and Sick Neonates, Chapter 7). These procedures are all safe if sterile equipment is used and meticulous aseptic techniques are practiced to minimize opportunities for microorganisms to invade the fragile host defenses of the newborn.

Although a pressure-monitoring system ideally should be a closed system, arterial cannulas frequently are also used for obtaining blood samples; these samples should be obtained aseptically with precautions to avoid contamination of the system. One source of contamination, for example, is ice used to chill syringes before obtaining the blood sample. Since some species of bacteria flourish in dextrose solutions at room temperature, this type of solution should not be used unless it is absolutely necessary.

Like all other intravascular cannulas, arterial cannulas may become colonized and serve as a nidus of infection. Percutaneous placement of peripheral arterial cannulas is associated with a lower risk of infection than is placement by surgical cutdown, however. Cannulas should remain at one site for no longer than 4 days and should be removed promptly if clinical signs suggest infection. A safe maximum duration of cannulation for umbilical arterial catheters has not been established. In general, intravascular catheters should not be used or left in place unless clearly indicated for medical management of the neonate. Guidelines for the prevention of infections associated with intravenous therapy and intravascular pressure monitoring have been published.

Total parenteral nutrition has been associated in the past with high rates of infection, including septicemia and fungemia. When properly administered, however, this technique is safe. A cooperative team approach between pharmacists, nurses, and physicians results in fewer infections and other complications and is strongly recommended. Meticulous attention should be paid to aseptic insertion and maintenance of the cannula and to techniques of fluid administration. All parenteral nutrition fluids should be compounded in a central pharmacy, preferably in a laminar flow hood. Because lipid emulsions are especially susceptible to contamination with a wide variety of bacterial and fungal pathogens that can proliferate to high concentrations within hours, particular caution must be taken in storage and administration of these emulsions. Unit-dose amounts may be delivered from the pharmacy; if bottles of emulsion are kept in the nursery refrigerator, care should be taken to prevent contamination. Opened bottles must be discarded no later than 24 hours after the seal has been broken.

Intravascular Flush Solutions

Solutions used for flushing intravascular catheters in neonates include sterile heparinized saline and dextrose. Those solutions available in the convenient multidose vials, however, are usually preserved with benzyl alcohol or a paraben. Since use of flush solutions preserved with benzyl alcohol has been associated with severe metabolic acidosis, clinical encephalopathy, and death in premature neonates, precautions should be taken to ensure that the solutions administered to neonates have not been preserved.

A system should be established with the hospital pharmacy to ensure a satisfactory and safe means of delivering the sterile, unpreserved fluids to the nursery areas. If heparin is used, it should be added to fluids in the hospital pharmacy whenever possible. To prevent problems from bacterial contamination of the unpreserved fluids, unit-dose amounts in syringes or a single container of fluid could be dispensed several times a day to the nursery; unused syringes or remaining fluid should be discarded when the new supply is received. Refrigeration will retard growth of most bacteria that may contaminate the solutions during preparation, and fluids should be refrigerated in the pharmacy once the seal of the container has been broken for admixture or unit-dose dispensing. Cold fluids should not be administered to neonates, however. It is important that flush solutions be kept at room temperature no longer than 8 hours before being used or discarded. Although numerous medications used for neonates are also preserved with benzyl alcohol or other agents, the volume of preservative received does not appear to be toxic if the neonates are not receiving intravascular flush solutions with preservatives.

Antibiotics for Neonates

Antibiotics, usually in combination, are commonly used for neonates in intensive care areas to treat presumed infections and to try to prevent infections in high-risk neonates who are undergoing multiple invasive procedures. Studies have not documented the efficacy of antibiotics used for prophylaxis, however; such use should be strongly discouraged. Topical antibiotics should be used only for very specific indications and on the order of a physician. The indiscriminate and inappropriate use of either systemic or topical antibiotics may result in the emergence of resistant strains of bacteria, making subsequent therapy of clinical infections more difficult and dangerous, and may alter the established flora of the neonate. In addition, systemic prophylactic therapy may partially suppress the clinical expression of infection, making diagnosis more difficult and delaying appropriate antimicrobial therapy.

If antibiotic therapy is essential for a neonate, appropriate specimens for culture should be obtained before the antibiotics are started. Broad spectrum coverage, such as that obtained with a penicillin and an aminoglycoside, is necessary. The newer broad spectrum drugs should be reserved for later therapy, if required, although as they are further evaluated for treatment of neonatal sepsis, meningitis, and other specific infections, recommendations for use will change. If the neonate improves and the results of cultures are not positive within 2–4 days, strong consideration should be given to stopping antibiotic therapy. If continued treatment for documented infection is indicated, the antibiotic should be changed, if necessary, to the most appropriate drug or drugs for the specific organism, its susceptibility, and the site of infection.

The relative frequencies of documented infection with different bacteria in neonates should be monitored by the infection control committee, along with the associated patterns of antimicrobial susceptibility. The most innocuous and specific antibiotic regimens should be selected after analysis of these data. For example, if kanamycin-resistant gram-negative bacteria only rarely cause infections during the first week of postnatal life but do cause infections more frequently in older infants, kanamycin could be used selectively in the younger group.

Skin Care of the Newborn

Risks and benefits of different skin care techniques for newborns should be considered, such as what effect the technique has on the skin itself, whether the agent used is absorbed and might be toxic, and whether the agent changes skin flora and might give rise to new infectious problems.

Currently available data suggest that the best method for managing the neonate's skin is to minimize manipulation with a technique known as dry skin care. The dry technique is recommended because (1) it reduces the neonate's heat loss by exposure, (2) it diminishes skin trauma, (3) it does not expose the neonate to agents with known or unknown side-effects, and (4) it requires less time.

Cleansing should be delayed until the neonate's temperature has stabilized. Sterile cotton sponges (not gauze) soaked with fresh water are used to remove blood and meconium from the face and head. Alternatively, a mild, nonmedicated soap, preferably in a single-use container or in a small bar reserved for a single neonate, can be used with careful water rinsing. The remainder of the neonate's skin may be left untouched unless it is grossly soiled. The vernix caseosa may have a protective function, although some believe it does not; there is no evidence to indicate it is harmful, however.

For the remainder of the neonate's stay in the hospital nursery, the buttocks and perianal regions should be cleansed with fresh water and cotton, with a mild soap and water at diaper changes, or as often as required.

Different antiseptic compounds for skin care have been studied for their effectiveness and safety in preventing colonization and infection in neonates. Hexachlorophene, which was widely used during the 1950s and 1960s, is relatively effective against gram-positive bacteria, particularly *S. aureus,* but it should not be used routinely for bathing neonates because it may be absorbed through intact skin and is potentially neurotoxic for neonates. Iodophors, although good antiseptics, have not been proved both safe and effective for routine skin care to prevent colonization and disease in newborns. The use of chlorhexidine gluconate, a compound that is poorly absorbed through intact skin, is under study.

No single method of cord care has proved superior in preventing colonization and disease. Methods presently used include local application of triple dye* and antimicrobial agents such as bacitracin or

---

*Triple dye is composed of 2.29 g brilliant green, 1.14 g proflavine hemisulfate, 2.29 g crystal violet, and enough water to make 1,000 ml. The skin absorption and toxicity of these agents in newborns have not been carefully studied.

silver sulfadiazine cream. Alcohol hastens drying of the cord, but, although frequently used as an antiseptic, probably is not effective in preventing cord colonization and omphalitis.

Immunization of Premature Neonates

The appropriate age for immunization of prematurely born neonates is uncertain. Few data are available on which to base firm recommendations. Common practice is to ignore gestational age and begin immunizations at the usual chronologic age, i.e., at 2 months of age, against diphtheria, tetanus, and pertussis (DTP) and polio. An infant who remains in the hospital longer than 2 months should be immunized with DTP according to the routine schedule for chronologic age, but polio vaccine should not be given to such an infant in order to avoid cross-infection in the nursery.

Isolation of Mothers and Neonates with Infections

Isolation procedures for patients with infectious diseases are intended to minimize or prevent the spread of microorganisms among patients, hospital personnel, and visitors. The revised system of patient isolation recommended for most hospitals in the United States is designed around seven basic categories:

1. Strict isolation
2. Respiratory isolation
3. Contact isolation
4. Drainage/secretion precautions
5. Enteric precautions
6. Blood/body fluid precautions
7. Tuberculosis isolation

Specific requirements for managing patients with infectious disease depend on the isolation category and the disease. Contact isolation is useful for patients with highly transmissible or epidemiologically important infections (e.g., patients colonized or infected with highly resistant bacteria) that do not require strict isolation. Drainage/secretion precautions are useful in managing patients with infectious discharge from wounds, lesions, and mucosal surfaces. Blood/body fluid precautions are intended for patients with infectious blood and/or body fluids, such as those with hepatitis B. Detailed descriptions of the isolation requirements are provided in *Guideline for Isolation Precau-*

tions in Hospitals* published by the Centers for Disease Control. The isolation categories were not designed for the special needs of neonates and nurseries, however, so that the specific procedures used within each category may need to be modified to manage neonates.

Obstetric patients with infections that may be transmitted to other patients or to medical or hospital personnel must be appropriately isolated. Frequently, this can be accomplished without requiring the patient to be in a private room or to move from the obstetric floor. It is essential to ensure that drainage or discharge from infectious lesions is adequately contained, that persons having contact with the infectious lesions use careful techniques (including, when appropriate, gown, gloves, and no-touch dressing change techniques), and that contaminated dressings, instruments, and other materials are appropriately discarded or wrapped before being sent for cleaning and disinfection or sterilization.

Isolation of Infected Postpartum Patients

Patients with group A streptococcal puerperal endometritis should be managed with contact isolation until 24 hours after initiation of adequate antimicrobial therapy; a private room is desirable, particularly if patient hygiene is poor. A gown and gloves should be used for direct contact with the infected area or drainage. Patients with abscesses or draining infections of the perineum or of abdominal wounds should also be managed with drainage/secretion precautions or, if necessary, contact isolation; a private room may be desirable.

Control measures essential for managing febrile puerperal patients are similar to those for managing patients with minor infections. Patients should be placed on drainage/secretion precautions; a private room is not essential. Careful attention to aseptic patient care techniques and meticulous hand-washing after contact with patients, especially after direct contact with infected areas, are essential. Gowns should be worn during direct patient contact and gloves used for contact with potentially infected areas or for changing dressings. Perineal pads, sanitary napkins, and dressings contaminated with potentially infectious drainage should be handled with instruments, promptly placed in double plastic bags, sealed, and incinerated. Contaminated instruments should be sealed in a plastic bag, labeled as contaminated, and sent for decontamination, cleaning, and sterilizing. Contaminated or potentially contaminated linen should be bagged, labeled, and handled appropriately.

---

*Formerly *Isolation Techniques in Hospitals.*

Postpartum patients with communicable diseases not unique to obstetric patients should be managed with appropriate precautions or isolation. If the risk of transmission to other patients is significant, or if the necessary procedures cannot be performed adequately on the obstetric unit, such a patient should be transferred to another nursing unit that can provide proper care.

Contact of Neonates with Their Infected Mothers

Since most maternal genital infections are caused by endogenous microorganisms that ascend into the uterus from the lower genital tract, postnatal spread of infection from this site to neonates is rare, except for group A streptococcal disease. Consequently, a febrile post-partum woman without a specific diagnosed site of infection usually may be allowed to handle and feed her newborn if she (1) is feeling well enough; (2) washes her hands thoroughly, under supervision; and (3) wears a clean hospital cover-gown to prevent contact of the baby with contaminated items, such a bedclothes, pads, and linen. A woman with communicable disease that is likely to be transmitted to her new-born should be separated from the newborn until the infection is no longer communicable.

A mother with a respiratory tract infection should be fully informed that transmission of such infections on hands or by fomites is common, and she should be instructed in careful hand-washing techniques and appropriate handling of tissues or other items contaminated with infectious secretions. It may be wise for her to use a surgical mask when she is with her newborn to reduce the chance of droplet spread of infection.

Breast-feeding is usually possible even if the mother has one of many different overt infections or if she is receiving antibiotics. Although antibiotics are secreted in breast milk in small amounts, this is usually not a contraindication to the continuation of breast-feeding.

Use of Cohorts for Infection Control

In large nurseries, cohorts of neonates may be established to minimize transmission of organisms or infectious diseases among different groups of neonates. A cohort usually consists of all well neonates born during the same 24- or 48-hour period; these neonates are kept in a single nursery room and, ideally, are cared for by a single group of personnel who do not care for any other cohort during a given shift. After the neonates in a cohort have been discharged, the room should be thoroughly cleaned and prepared to accept the next cohort.

The use of cohorts is not practical as a routine for small nurseries or for those facilities with intensive care and graded care units. Even in these facilities, however, this approach can be useful in efforts to control epidemics or in the management of a group of neonates colonized or infected with a specific microbial strain. Although separate rooms for these cohorts are ideal, they are not mandatory if a means is devised to demarcate cohort lines within a single large room and if personnel assigned to a cohort provide care only for neonates in that cohort.

During an epidemic, neonates with overt infection and those who are colonized must be identified rapidly and placed in cohorts. If rapid identification of these neonates is not possible, exposed neonates should be placed in a cohort separate from those with disease, from unexposed neonates, and from newly admitted neonates. The success of cohort programs depends largely on the willingness and ability of nursery and ancillary personnel to adhere strictly to the cohort system and to follow established patient care practices.

Neonates with Suspected or Proved Infections

Previous recommendations for handling infected or possibly infected neonates were based on two assumptions: (1) segregation by removal to a geographically isolated room was necessary for the protection of uninfected neonates, and (2) the isolated neonate would be under close scrutiny and, therefore, would receive better care. Neither of these assumptions is completely correct.

The housing of an infected neonate depends on the overall condition of the neonate and the type of care required, the available space and facilities, the nurse/patient ratio, and the size and type of the newborn service. Other factors to be considered include the type of infection (specific viral or bacterial pathogen), the clinical manifestations, the source and possible modes of spread of the infection, and the number of colonized or infected neonates.

Isolation rooms are unnecessary for many infected neonates if the following conditions are met: (1) sufficient nursing and medical staff (see Chapter 3) are on duty to provide comprehensive care, (2) sufficient space is available for a 4- to 6-ft aisle or area between neonatal stations, (3) two or more sinks for hand-washing are available in each nursery room or area, (4) continuing instruction is provided about the ways in which infections spread. If these criteria are not met, an isolation room with separate scrub facilities is necessary.

It has often been assumed that forced air incubators provide adequate isolation for infected neonates. These incubators filter incoming air but not the air that is discharged into the nursery. They are satisfactory, therefore, for limited protective isolation of neonates but should not be relied upon to prevent transmission of microorganisms from infected neonates to others. Furthermore, the surfaces of incubators housing neonates are readily contaminated with organisms infecting or colonizing the neonates, and the hands and forearms of personnel working with the neonates through portholes are likely to be colonized.

Specific management of neonates with suspected or definite infections varies somewhat from nursery to nursery. For optimal management of neonates with each type of infection, hospitals should have written procedures appropriate to the facilities and staff available. To minimize the risk of additional infections, each instance of infectious disease should be investigated as to etiology, probable source of infection, and mode of spread.

Neonates that are at higher risk of developing an infection are those born (1) under conditions in which they are exposed to an environment heavily contaminated with microorganisms, (2) to mothers with membranes ruptured for 24 hours or more, or (3) to mothers suspected of harboring or incubating infectious disease. These neonates require early diagnosis and treatment of infection to prevent transmission of infection (or colonizing microorganisms) to other neonates in the nursery. Given satisfactory conditions in the nursery, the neonates may be cared for in the admission/observation area or in the regular newborn care area.

Blood and cerebrospinal fluid cultures should be performed on neonates delivered after prolonged rupture of membranes if (1) their mothers have had any suggestion of chorioamnionitis, or (2) findings in the neonates themselves (including the need for special resuscitative procedures) can be interpreted as infection. Cultures from skin and mucosal surfaces, or urine or gastric aspirates, are not recommended routinely because positive cultures from these sites do not necessarily indicate those pathogens that are causing systemic disease. Specific specimens required for culture should be determined by the clinical condition of the neonate. Those who were delivered after prolonged rupture of membranes but who have no signs that suggest infection and whose mothers have no signs or symptoms that suggest infection should be observed carefully; the need for cultures should be determined by the clinical condition of these neonates.

NEONATES WITH SEVERE BACTERIAL INFECTION. Under ideal conditions, neonates with septicemia, bacterial meningitis, or pneumonia present little additional risk of infection to other neonates. To receive satisfactory care, these neonates should be treated in the intensive care unit.

NEONATES WITH GASTROENTERITIS OR DRAINING LESIONS. Ideally, neonates with gastroenteritis (diarrhea), draining lesions (e.g., caused by *S. aureus*), or purulent conjunctivitis should be placed in a separate or isolation room. They may be treated in the general intensive or intermediate care areas provided that these areas are adequately staffed and have sufficient space and equipment to allow isolation and proper care. Neonates with these infections may also be cared for in newborn nurseries, although housing the infected neonates in a separate room or observation area is desirable. The most important factor in preventing the spread of infection is to provide sufficient nursing personnel to care for the neonates. If more than one neonate is infected, a cohort approach should be taken.

Enteric precautions or drainage/secretion precautions should be observed, as appropriate. A gown and disposable gloves should be used for providing direct patient care, particularly for changing diapers or dressings or for direct contact with the infected area. Contaminated items must be disposed of properly. It must be emphasized that the environment surrounding neonates with these infections may be heavily contaminated with the infecting microorganism.

NEONATES WITH CONGENITAL INFECTIONS. Those neonates who have congenital infections such as cytomegalovirus, rubella, and syphilis may be highly infectious. Depending on the infection, neonates may excrete high titers of the infectious agent in urine, from the nasopharynx, and from mucous membrane or cutaneous lesions; duration of excretion is variable, but it may be prolonged for months in some cases. Neonates with asymptomatic or mild infections frequently excrete the infectious agent.

Neonates with these congenital infections should be physically segregated (a private room may be desirable) and managed with drainage/secretion precautions. Hand-washing, particularly after changing diapers, should be thorough; gowns and disposable gloves may be desirable for direct patient contact.

Neonates with congenital toxoplasmosis need not be isolated.

NEONATES WITH VIRAL INFECTIONS. Many viruses, such as respiratory syncytial virus, coxsackieviruses, or echoviruses, spread rapidly among neonates and personnel in a nursery; such infections can be serious in the neonates and sometimes result in death. Neonates may have prolonged asymptomatic shedding of selected viruses after resolution of the clinical illness, thus becoming a reservoir of infection. The viruses are believed to be transmitted predominantly by direct or indirect contact on contaminated hands of personnel or by contaminated environmental surfaces or fomites. Contact isolation may be required to prevent this type of spread, but specific requirements vary with the infecting virus. For example, respiratory syncytial virus is shed primarily from the respiratory tract, while coxsackieviruses or echoviruses can be shed from the throat or stool.

Airborne Transmission of Infection

Under most circumstances, neonates are relatively ineffective disseminators of infectious bacterial or viral aerosols that could spread infection by air. Neonates with definite or possible infections caused by a viral agent that could be transmitted by the airborne route should be separated from other neonates (1) by enclosing all other neonates in the area in forced draft incubators (i.e., reverse isolation), (2) by rooming-in of the neonate and mother, or (3) by transfer of the neonate from the nursery area.

SPECIFIC INFECTIOUS PROBLEMS DURING PREGNANCY AND MANAGEMENT OF THE NEWBORN

Collectively, infections are one of the most common problems confronting obstetricians. Bacteria, mycoplasma, *Chlamydia*, and viruses all may cause disease in the pregnant woman; many of the infections are subclinical and require serologic or other laboratory tests for detection. Certain infections that occur antepartum or intrapartum may have a significant effect on the fetus and newborn; proper management of the mother during pregnancy and at delivery and of the newborn postnatally can prevent or modify many of the serious problems and can minimize risk of subsequent transmission of infection in the nursery. Close communication and cooperation among all perinatal personnel are essential to obtain the best results.

Gonorrhea

Maternal Infection

Gonorrhea is most often an asymptomatic infection during pregnancy. Although salpingitis is rare in pregnancy, disseminated gonococcal disease (e.g., with rash, fever, and arthritis) may occur more frequently during pregnancy. Gonococcal infections in pregnant women, even though asymptomatic, may be associated with an increased incidence of perinatal morbidity and mortality, including fetal wastage, early and prolonged rupture of membranes, premature labor, and delivery of low-birth-weight neonates. The incidence of complications appears to be particularly high in women with intrapartum gonococcal infection. This infection may result in fetal sepsis or scalp abscess if intrauterine fetal monitoring is used.

In order to prevent gonococcal infection in neonates, cervical cultures should be obtained during pregnancy from mothers who are at high risk of infection. Infected women should be treated, and their newborns should be provided with appropriate prophylaxis or treatment. In high-risk populations, endocervical cultures for gonococci should be taken during the first prenatal visit, and a second culture should be taken late in the third trimester (see Chapter 4). Drug regimens of choice are those for uncomplicated gonorrhea, except that tetracycline should not be used because of its potential toxic effects for mother and fetus. Women allergic to penicillin or probenicid should be treated with spectinomycin. Women with gonococcal infection at delivery should be managed with drainage/secretion precautions until effective systemic therapy has been administered for 24 hours.

Gonococcal and Other Infections in Newborns

The prevalence of largely asymptomatic genital gonococcal infection in pregnant women and the occurrence of gonococcal ophthalmia in approximately 28% of untreated neonates born to infected women indicate the need for prophylaxis for all neonates. A 1% silver nitrate solution in single-dose ampules or a sterile ophthalmic ointment containing tetracycline (1%) or erythromycin (0.5%) in single-use tubes are acceptable regimens for prophylaxis of gonococcal ophthalmia neonatorum. Erythromycin ointment may also be effective prophylaxis for neonatal ophthalmia caused by *Chlamydia trachomatis*, although its use for this purpose does not reduce the frequency of chlamydial infection at other sites (see Appendix E).

None of the agents used for prophylaxis should be flushed from the eye after instillation. Critical studies have not evaluated the efficacy of silver nitrate prophylaxis with and without flushing, but anecdotal reports suggest that flushing may reduce the prophylactic effectiveness of the drug. In addition, flushing probably does not reduce the incidence of chemical conjuctivitis.

Prophylaxis should be given as soon after birth as practical. Although definitive data are not available, delaying prophylaxis for up to 1 hour after birth probably does not affect efficacy and may facilitate initial maternal-neonatal attachment. Hospitals in which prophylaxis is delayed should establish a check system to ensure that all neonates are treated.

Neonates born by cesarean delivery should also receive prophylaxis against gonococcal ophthalmia. Although gonococcal infection is usually transmitted during passage through the birth canal, neonates may have been infected by ascending organisms. The precise risk of gonococcal infection in untreated neonates born by cesarean delivery has not been determined.

Neonates born to mothers with recognized gonococcal infection should receive a single injection of aqueous crystalline penicillin G, 50,000 units for full-term or 20,000 units for low-birth-weight neonates. Topical prophylaxis alone is inadequate for these neonates.

Neonates with clinical ophthalmia or complicated (disseminated) gonococcal infection should be hospitalized and treated with aqueous crystalline penicillin G, 50,000 units/kg body weight daily in two doses administered intravenously for 7 days. Gonococcal ophthalmia is highly contagious, and infected neonates should be managed with contact isolation (it is especially important that gloves be used for contact with the infected area) for 24 hours after treatment is initiated. The eyes should be irrigated with saline. Topical antibiotics are superfluous when appropriate systemic antibiotic therapy is given. Ophthalmologic consultation is suggested.

Neonates with extraocular gonococcal infections, such as arthritis, septicemia, or meningitis, require more intensive treatment.

Some strains of *Neisseria gonorrhoeae* may be resistant to penicillin. Attempts should be made to isolate the organism from both mother and child, and the antimicrobial susceptibility of all isolates should be determined. Susceptibilities would then be available as a therapeutic guide should other forms of antimicrobial therapy become necessary because of poor clinical response to penicillin.

Herpes Simplex Infection

Maternal Infection and Management of Delivery

Herpes genitalis, caused by HSV, is characterized by multiple, painful vesicles and ulcers in various stages. Many HSV infections are subclinical, however, and women with genital cultures positive for the virus are frequently asymptomatic.

Primary genital HSV infection, either type I or II, during pregnancy may be associated with spontaneous abortion, preterm delivery, and, rarely, congenital anomalies. Newborns delivered of women with genital herpes are at risk of developing herpes infection, with death or severe neurologic sequelae common in those affected. The risk of infection in the newborn appears to be highest with primary genital infection of the pregnant woman, but transmission also occurs with recurrent maternal infection. As many as 70% of women with neonates who develop HSV infection are asymptomatic at time of delivery.

It is essential, therefore, to inform pregnant women about the ways in which infection can be avoided, to screen pregnant women selectively for this infection, and to perform cesarean delivery in patients with evidence of active herpes infection. Women should be counseled to avoid sexual contact, including oral-genital contact, during the last several months of pregnancy if their partners have genital HSV infection.

Women with a history of recurrent genital HSV infection, those with active disease during the current pregnancy, and those whose sexual partners have proved genital HSV infection should be monitored with virologic or cytologic studies, or both, at least twice during the last 6 weeks of pregnancy. It is important to emphasize that clinical examination may be unrevealing in patients with documented infection. Papanicolaou smears of the cervix can be obtained in most clinical facilities, but will identify HSV-infected women on only three-quarters of virologically proved cases. While at the present time isolation of HSV in cell culture is the most sensitive and accurate method, other methods of monitoring women by virus identification in cervical smears stained with fluorescein-tagged or enzyme-linked HSV antibody are being evaluated. Serologic tests are not useful for screening and management.

The risk of neonatal infection is as high as 40%–50% in neonates born vaginally to women who are culture-positive at delivery, to those with primary genital infections, and to those whose fetal membranes have been ruptured for longer than 4–6 hours, particularly those with membranes ruptured for longer than 24 hours before delivery. Fetal scalp electrode monitoring may result in direct inoculation of HSV from maternal infection, even if the mother is asymptomatic.

Management of each delivery must be based on the probability of HSV infection of the neonate, the status of the fetal membranes, the length of gestation, and the risk of cesarean delivery. A woman is considered free of infection and may be delivered vaginally if virologic or cytologic test results are negative on two successive examinations, the last of which was obtained within 1 week of delivery, and clinical lesions are not detected at delivery. If a woman at term has genital HSV infection as indicated by clinical findings or, preferably, cytologic or virologic studies, a cesarean delivery should be performed before onset of labor and rupture of membranes. If the fetal membranes have been ruptured for less than 6 hours, there may be some benefit from cesarean delivery; conversely, there is no apparent advantage to cesarean delivery if the membranes have been ruptured for more than 24 hours. If the duration of membrane rupture is unknown for a woman in labor who had confirmed genital herpes at 32 weeks' gestation or later, management should be based on the best assessment of the relative risks. These recommendations, although widely followed, are based on relatively few well-studied cases. The results of these studies suggest that cesarean delivery significantly reduces the risk of HSV infection to the newborn but does not eliminate it.

Women with genital herpetic infection can be managed safely with drainage/secretion precautions in all areas of labor and delivery and on the postpartum unit; those with severe primary infection should be managed with contact isolation in private rooms. Personnel and the patient should use gloves for direct contact with the infected area or for handling contaminated dressings, and meticulous hand-washing should be emphasized. Labor and delivery rooms require only routine, careful cleaning and disinfection before being used by another patient.

Management of Exposed Newborns

Most neonates who develop HSV infection acquire their infection perinatally from their mothers. Onset of infection may occur at any time during the first month. The average age of onset is 6 days for generalized disease, 11 days for central nervous system disease. About 70% of neonates with HSV infection develop vesicular skin lesions as an early manifestation; diagnosis of the disease in neonates without skin lesions is difficult and requires a high index of suspicion to request appropriate tests. Asymptomatic infection of newborns has been documented only rarely.

Because HSV infection has occasionally been transmitted among neonates in nurseries and because this infection is potentially severe in newborns, precautions should be taken to minimize the risk of transmission within the nursery. Experts disagree about the precise precautions required, however. It is generally agreed that a neonate born by vaginal delivery to a woman with active genital HSV infection should be segregated from other neonates, although an isolation room is not essential. Personnel working with the infected neonate should wash their hands meticulously after caring for the neonate and use techniques that prevent transmission of any virus that might be shed during the later incubation or early clinical states of disease. Viral cultures, liver function studies, and cerebrospinal fluid examination of the neonate should be done. To allow early detection of disease, it may be necessary to observe the neonate in the hospital for up to 2 weeks.

A neonate born by cesarean delivery before rupture of the membranes is at minimal risk of developing HSV infection and can be managed with few special precautions. The neonate should be observed in the hospital for several days and followed closely after discharge; the mother should be instructed to observe the neonate carefully for any early sign of infection.

Early signs of HSV infection in newborns are frequently nonspecific and subtle. Neonates known to have been exposed to HSV who develop any signs of illness compatible with HSV infection should be managed as though they had HSV infection until proved otherwise. They should be physically segregated and managed with contact isolation; an isolation room is desirable. Personnel having contact with skin lesions or potentially infectious secretions should use gowns and gloves. Neonates with HSV disease should be managed in a facility that provides Level III care, and expert consultation about recommended antiviral drug therapy should be sought.

Contact of Neonates with Their HSV-Infected Mothers

A mother with HSV infection should be instructed about her infection and taught hygienic measures to prevent postnatal transmission of HSV infection. Before touching her newborn, the mother should don a clean gown and wash her hands carefully. If the mother has genital herpes infection, her newborn may room-in with her after she has been taught protective measures; this may be an effective method of segregating the exposed neonate from others in the nursery. Breast-feeding is permissible if the mother has no vesicular herpetic lesions in the area and all active cutaneous lesions are covered. A mother with herpes labialis (cold sore) or stomatitis should wear a disposable surgical mask when touching her newborn until the lesions have crusted and dried. She should not kiss or nuzzle her newborn until the lesions have cleared. Direct contact of a newborn with other family members or friends who have active HSV infection should be avoided.

Rubella

Prevention and Management of Infection During Pregnancy

Surveillance for susceptibility to rubella infection is essential for good prenatal care. Each patient should be screened serologically at the first prenatal visit unless she is proved to be immune by previous serologic test or documented vaccination. Immunity is most commonly determined by the hemagglutination inhibition (HAI) test; in a properly controlled test, any detectable antibody indicates immunity. Seropositive women do not need further testing, regardless of subsequent history of exposure. Repeat titers should be obtained from seronegative patients who have been exposed to rubella or whose physical findings suggest infection. Specimens should be obtained as soon as possible after exposure, again 2 weeks later, and, if necessary, 4 weeks after exposure. Acute and convalescent sera specimens should be tested on the same day in the same laboratory; a fourfold or greater rise in titer or seroconversion indicates acute infection. Rubella-specific IgM testing or isolation of virus from throat swabs rapidly establishes a diagnosis of acute rubella if the tests are available.

If rubella is diagnosed in a pregnant woman, the patient should be advised of the risk of delivering a neonate with congenital rubella syndrome. Therapeutic abortion should be offered as an option. Limited data indicate that the administration of immune globulin (IG), 0.55 ml/kg, as soon as possible after exposure may prevent or modify infection in exposed susceptible persons. The absence of clinical signs in a woman who has received IG does not guarantee that infection has been prevented, however; neonates with congenital rubella syndrome have been born to mothers given IG shortly after exposure. If termination of pregnancy is not an option, administration of IG as soon as possible after exposure should be considered.

For rubella-susceptible women of reproductive age, vaccination is available; the RA 27/3 vaccine is highly effective and has few side-effects. An excellent time to vaccinate susceptible women is the puerperium. Prevaccination serologic testing for susceptibility is not mandatory and should not impede vaccination. Receipt of RhIG or blood products is not a contraindication to vaccination, but serologic testing should be done 6–8 weeks postvaccination to confirm seroconversion.

Vaccinated women, including those vaccinated during the puerperium, should be warned to avoid conception for 3 months. Available data suggest that vaccine virus is considerably less teratogenic than is wild virus, but data are not sufficient to define the risk precisely. A woman who conceives within 3 months of rubella vaccination or is inadvertently vaccinated in early pregnancy should be informed about a possible injury to the fetus. To assist with developing firm recommendations for management of this problem, physicians caring for a pregnant woman inadvertently immunized with rubella vaccine should report the case as soon as possible to the Centers for Disease Control through the state health department.

Management of Exposed or Infected Neonates

Neonates who are suspected of having congenital rubella infection or who were born to women known to have had rubella during pregnancy should be housed in a private room and managed with contact isolation. Care should be provided only by personnel known to be immune to rubella. They should wear a gown and gloves while providing direct care and wash their hands carefully after caring for the neonate or handling diapers or other contaminated items; a mask is not required.

Every effort should be made to isolate the virus from the neonate and to document the infection. Neonates with congenital rubella should be considered contagious up to 1 year of age unless virus cultures are negative. Cases of congenital rubella syndrome or birth defects believed to be caused by rubella infection should be reported to the state health department.

Hepatitis Infections

Management of Maternal Hepatitis Type B Infection

Hepatitis B virus (HBV) infection in a pregnant woman may result in severe disease for the mother and chronic infection in the newborn (see nomenclature in Table 6–1). Transmission of HBV from mother to neonate apparently occurs most often during delivery. Neonates born to mothers who have HBV during the last trimester of pregnancy or during the postpartum period are at high risk of acquiring infection. Pregnancy is not a contraindication to the use of inactivated HBV vaccine in women who are at high risk of HBV infection.

Neonates born to mothers who are chronic carriers of hepatitis B antigen (HBsAG) are at variable risk of developing infection; studies in the United States have shown a low risk of transmission to the neonate, but those from Asia have shown a high risk. Factors that

Table 6–1. *Hepatitis Type B Nomenclature*

Abbreviation	Term	Comments
HBV	Hepatitis B virus	Etiologic agent of hepatitis type B (previously "serum" or "long incubation" hepatitis); also known as Dane particle.
HBsAg	Hepatitis B surface antigen	Surface antigen(s) of HBV, detectable in large quantity in serum; several subtypes identified.
HBeAg	Hepatitis B e antigen	Soluble antigen; correlates with HBV replication, high titer HBV in serum, and infectivity of serum.
HBcAg	Hepatitis B core antigen	No commercial test available.
Anti-HBs	Antibody to HBsAg	Indicates past infection with and immunity to HBV, passive antibody from HBIG, or immune response from HBV vaccine.
Anti-HBe	Antibody to HBeAg	Presence in serum of HBsAg carrier suggests low titer of HBV.
Anti-HBc	Antibody to HBcAg	Indicates past infection with HBV at some undefined time.
HBIG	Hepatitis B immune globulin	

increase the risk of transmission from mothers to neonates are a high maternal titer of HBsAg and presence of e antigen (HBeAg). Approximately 80% of neonates born to HBeAg-positive mothers become infected, and most become chronic carriers. Mothers with antibody against HBeAg are unlikely to transmit HBV infection to their newborns.

Pregnant women who are likely to be chronic HBsAg carriers, especially those who are of Asian origin or who abuse drugs, should be screened for HBsAg. Women in high-risk groups may also be screened for HBeAg. Chronic carriers of HBsAg should be managed in the office or clinic and hospital with blood/body fluid precautions. Labor, delivery, and nursery personnel should be notified in advance of anticipated delivery and arrangements to have hepatitis B immune globulin (HBIG) available at delivery should be made. Precautions must be taken to prevent transmission of HBV infection to hospital personnel during the labor, delivery, and postpartum periods.

Management of Newborns Exposed to HBV

Neonates infected at birth with HBV frequently become chronic carriers of HBsAg and have a high frequency of serious chronic sequelae; therefore, every effort should be made to prevent infection.

The neonates should be bathed carefully as soon as possible after birth to remove maternal blood and secretions that contaminated their skin during birth. Personnel who handle the blood-contaminated neonates are advised to wear gloves to protect themselves. After being bathed, the neonates may be managed without special precautions for the remainder of their stay in the nursery. Neonates and mothers may have normal contact, or they may room-in (see Chapter 7 for recommendations on breast-feeding). The neonates should be carefully examined and tested periodically during their first year of life to determine whether they have become chronic carriers of HBsAg.

The administration of HBIG reduces the rate of HBV infection in neonates; comparisons with general immune globulin (IG) have not been made. Neonates born to mothers with acute hepatitis B or those who are HBsAg-positive (regardless of HBeAg status) should be given an injection of HBIG, 0.5 ml intramuscularly, as soon as possible after birth, preferably within 1 hour. To avoid inoculation of virus contaminating the skin, the injection site should be thoroughly cleaned before administration of HBIG (or other agents). Additional injections of HBIG should be administered to these children at 3 and 6 months of age. Recommendations on the number and timing of doses of HBIG may change as additional experience is acquired.

Since children whose mothers are chronic HBsAg carriers will be continuously exposed to HBV throughout their childhood, they should also receive inactivated HBV vaccine. The optimum timing for vaccination in conjunction with HBIG administration has not been established. Pending additional information, it is recommended that the series of three vaccinations begin at 3 months of age or shortly thereafter. Studies are being conducted to determine the immunogenicity and efficacy of vaccine at birth, with or without HBIG.

Management of Newborns Exposed to Hepatitis A Virus

Ordinarily, neonates of mothers who have hepatitis type A infection during pregnancy should not receive IG. Neonates born to mothers with hepatitis A infection at delivery or during the postpartum period should receive 0.02 ml/kg IG intramuscularly at birth or as soon as maternal infection is diagnosed; protection for the neonates is uncertain.

In the nursery, the neonates should be bathed carefully but do not need other special precautions.

Group B β-Hemolytic *Streptococcus* Colonization and Disease

The proportion of pregnant women and neonates colonized with group B β-hemolytic streptococci ranges from approximately 5%–

35%. Group B streptococci (types Ia, Ib, Ic, II, III) are important causes of disease in the neonate and infant. In women, the organism occasionally causes significant postpartum infection, but rectal or genital carriage is usually asymptomatic. Infection is frequently transmitted from the mother to the newborn, either in utero or intrapartum; nosocomial acquisition by the neonate (probably neonate to neonate via the hands of personnel) also occurs. Neonatal group B streptococcal disease has an incidence of 1/1000 live births, although the incidence varies widely among hospitals. Early onset disease occurs in about 1 infant per 100 colonized women.

No recommendations can be made at present about treatment to eradicate group B streptococcal colonization of mothers, neonates, or nursery personnel, since treatment has not been demonstrated to reduce either maternal or neonatal disease and extensive culturing is required to identify those who are colonized. Studies of the effectiveness of penicillin G administered to colonized pregnant women at delivery or to neonates in the delivery room are in progress; published reports indicate varying results. Currently, chemoprophylaxis should be considered for investigational purposes only.

Neonates with group B streptococcal disease can be treated in the intensive care area if routine precautions are taken to prevent transmission of bacterial infection. In view of the high percentage of colonized neonates within many nurseries and the lack of effective means to eradicate colonization, routine identification and isolation of asymptomatic carriers are impractical. Other methods of control (e.g., treatment of asymptomatic carriers with penicillin or treatment of the umbilical cord with triple dye or hexachlorophene) have also proved to be impractical or unreliable.

Detection of a nosocomial problem caused by group B *Streptococcus* is difficult because most neonates have late onset disease days or weeks after discharge from the nursery. If a cluster of cases occurs in neonates born at a single hospital, however, an investigation is warranted. Establishing a cohort of neonates in the nursery may be a useful control measure. Meticulous hand-washing by all personnel, sufficient personnel on all shifts, and adequate spacing between neonates may be important in limiting neonate-to-neonate transmission within the nursery.

Cytomegalovirus Infections

Cytomegalovirus is a ubiquitous virus that causes infection of little direct concern to healthy adults. The epidemiology of infection is not completely known, and many questions remain unanswered. Primary maternal cytomegalovirus infection early in pregnancy may result in a congenitally diseased neonate. Reactivation of latent cytomegalovirus infection is relatively common during pregnancy and may result in congenital infection of a neonate. Although most such infections are clinically inapparent at birth, late sequelae may occur. Infected mothers also may excrete the virus in their breast milk, and infection can be acquired postnatally, although most occur without clinical manifestations.

No specific recommendations can be made to prevent primary cytomegalovirus infections of pregnant women. Avoiding intimate contact with known infected persons may be useful, since transmission of the virus most often appears to be by direct contact. Good personal hygiene is probably important in preventing infection.

Neonates known or suspected to have cytomegalovirus infection may excrete virus in urine and respiratory secretions; drainage/secretion precautions may be indicated for managing these neonates. Personnel should wash their hands carefully after providing care for the neonate or handling contaminated objects, particularly diapers.

Neonates of seronegative mothers are at risk of severe morbidity or death if they acquire cytomegalovirus infection. These infections can be transmitted to neonates by transfusion of blood from seropositive donors or by ingestion of cytomegalovirus-contaminated milk from milk banks. Research data suggest that screening donor blood for antibody against cytomegalovirus may reduce morbidity from transfusion in premature neonates.

Tuberculosis

Maternal Infection

Although tuberculosis occurs infrequently in most obstetric populations, prenatal visits have traditionally been a time to perform skin testing for infection with tuberculosis. This screening test is especially important for populations at high risk of infection and in areas with high endemic rates of this disease. In patients with a positive skin test for tuberculosis, a chest x-ray film should be obtained to rule out active disease. The course of the disease is not altered by pregnancy, although the clinical condition may be exacerbated during the puerperium.

Because of the social environment in which tuberculosis occurs and the risk of significant morbidity and mortality to the newborn from the disease, the local health department should be notified about a suspected or documented case in a pregnant woman, a new mother, or her family. A thorough family study should be conducted to determine if others in contact with the mother or neonate are infected. Treatment should be initiated for anyone found to be infected and continuing care arranged.

A pregnant patient with active tuberculosis should be managed as other patients with tuberculosis are managed. Sputum specimens for mycobacterial culture should be obtained, and antimicrobial susceptibilities to the primary drugs should be determined. Since experience during pregnancy with the newer antituberculosis drugs is limited, isoniazid and ethambutol are recommended. Pregnant patients who are receiving isoniazid also should be given vitamin B_6 (50 mg daily) to avoid interference with pyridoxine metabolism.

Prophylactic therapy with isoniazid may be indicated for selected patients. Because of its potential hepatotoxicity, its use for prophylaxis should be restricted to those whose skin test results have become positive within the past 2 years or those who live in a household with a person who has active disease. Initiation of isoniazid prophylaxis can usually be deferred until the second trimester; it can be deferred until after delivery if the woman's positive reaction to the tuberculin skin test is first discovered during the third trimester. Therapy should be continued for 1 year after delivery.

Management of Exposed Newborns

The care of neonates born to mothers with tuberculosis should be individualized. Tuberculosis in neonates appears to result most commonly from airborne infection during the perinatal and postnatal periods; mothers with active but undiagnosed and untreated infections are a frequent source. Congenital tuberculosis (transplacental infection) is rare, but, when it occurs, results in severe disease with high mortality. Establishing a definitive diagnosis of tuberculosis in a newborn is frequently difficult. Therapy often must be initiated on the basis of clinical judgment and a high index of suspicion.

A healthy neonate born to a woman with tuberculosis that is active or of unknown infectiousness can be managed routinely without special precautions in the nursery. The neonate must be separated from the mother at birth, however, and kept separated until the neonate has developed adequate resistance and the mother is bacteriologically noninfective. The neonate should be placed on isoniazid prophylactic therapy and can be returned to the mother after she has begun chemotherapy and has negative sputum cultures. The mother and neonate should be followed carefully.

BCG vaccine is suggested for a neonate who is skin test–negative but is in a household with untreated or ineffectively treated individuals who have sputum-positive pulmonary tuberculosis. Neonates given BCG should not receive isoniazid and should be separated from their mothers or other potentially contagious individuals until they become tuberculin skin test–positive.

Syphilis

Pregnant women should be screened with a serologic test for syphilis at the first prenatal visit and after exposure to an infected partner, and late in the third trimester or at delivery. A repeat test for syphilis or other sexually transmitted diseases should be performed if the patient belongs to a high-risk population. Serologic and other appropriate diagnostic tests should be performed if suspicious lesions develop. Hematogenous transplacental infection of the fetus is the most common means of transmission of congenital syphilis, although direct contact of the neonate with infectious lesions during or after birth can also result in infection. Transplacental infection can occur throughout pregnancy and during any stage of maternal infection.

Pregnant women with syphilis should be treated with standard regimens for acquired primary, secondary, or early latent syphilis if they are not allergic to penicillin. Patients allergic to penicillin should be treated with erythromycin in a dose schedule appropriate for recently acquired syphilis in nonpregnant patients. This regimen is safe for both mother and fetus, but its efficacy has not been adequately documented. Neonates born after treatment of the mother with this regimen should be examined for congenital syphilis; examination of the cerebrospinal fluid should be included. Tetracycline and the estolate ester of erythromycin should not be used in pregnant women because of potential toxic effects.

Results of the maternal serologic tests and treatment, if given, should be recorded in the neonate's medical record or be made available to the neonate's physician. A serologic test for syphilis should be performed on cord or venous blood of neonates for whom the results of maternal tests or treatment are unavailable or questionable.

A diagnosis of congenital syphilis frequently is difficult to establish since clinical evidence of infection may not be apparent at birth and serologic tests may be difficult to interpret. Neonates with a positive result on a serologic test for syphilis or a history of partial or questionably adequate maternal treatment for infection must be followed carefully. A reactive VDRL test for syphilis or fluorescent treponemal antibody–absorption (FTA–ABS) test on cord or neonatal blood does not necessarily indicate the neonate is infected. If the reaction is caused by passively transferred antibody, the reactivity should decline and the test result be negative when the infant is 3–4 months of age. A persistently reactive serologic test for syphilis suggests infection and a rising titer is almost diagnostic. The IgM–FTA–ABS test is more specific for diagnosis for congenital syphilis, and a positive test result is highly significant; a negative test result, however, does not exclude active infection in the neonate.

Moist, open syphilitic lesions are infectious. Drainage/secretion precautions and blood/body fluid precautions should be used for a neonate suspected of having congenital syphilis. Health care personnel (and parents) should wear gloves when handling the neonate until appropriate antibiotic therapy has been administered for at least 24 hours. Individuals who have had close contact with the neonate before isolation precautions and treatment were instituted should be examined clinically and tested serologically for infection.

Varicella-Zoster (Chickenpox)

Women with varicella during pregnancy are usually no more severely ill than other adults; they should be followed closely, however, as fatalities have been reported. Varicella during early pregnancy is occasionally associated with congenital malformations or fetal mortality. If onset of clinical maternal infection occurs in the last 4 days of pregnancy, subsequent infection in the newborn may be fulminant, with systemic and neurologic involvement and death. Varicella-zoster immune globulin (VZIG), available from the regional blood centers of the American Red Cross Blood Services, should be administered to newborns of mothers who have onset of varicella within 5 days before delivery or 48 hours after delivery. If administered promptly, VZIG is most protective.

Women with varicella must be kept in strict isolation if admitted to a hospital. Neonates exposed in utero or postnatally to varicella should be segregated and managed expectantly during the incubation period. Those neonates with varicella infection should be isolated in a private room and managed with strict isolation for the duration of illness. Neonates with congenital varicella do not need to be managed with special precautions.

Toxoplasmosis

Caused by the protozoan parasite *Toxoplasma gondii*, toxoplasmosis is usually an asymptomatic or mild, nonspecific illness resembling infectious mononucleosis when it is acquired by older children or adults. Congenital toxoplasmosis, however, ranges from asymptomatic infection to severe infection with death. Clinical manifestations of fetal infection include prematurity, intrauterine growth retardation, encephalitis, microcephaly or hydrocephalus, and chorioretinitis. Sur vivors may have severe sequelae.

Humans acquire toxoplasmosis by consuming poorly cooked meat or by ingesting sporulated oocysts excreted in cat feces. Congenital toxoplasmosis results from acute infection of the pregnant woman. Infection acquired during the first trimester is apparently associated with a lower rate of congenital infection, but the majority of the infected neonates are severely affected. Conversely, maternal infection during the third trimester results in a high rate of congenital infection, but the majority of affected neonates have asymptomatic infection.

The primary diagnostic tests for toxoplasmosis are serologic; results must be interpreted carefully. Seroconversion or a fourfold or greater rise in IgG antibody titer on serial specimens tested simultaneously suggest recent infection. IgM-specific antibodies can be detected by enzyme-linked immunosorbent assay or immunofluorescence.

Congenital toxoplasmosis can be averted by preventing acute infection in pregnant women. Only thoroughly cooked meats should be eaten. Cat litter should be disposed of daily (oocysts are not infective during the first 24 hours after passage), or cats should be avoided. Domestic cats should be fed only commercially prepared cat food and should not be allowed to hunt wild rodents or eat raw or partially cooked meat and kitchen scraps. Pregnant women with negative or unknown *Toxoplasma* titers should avoid gardening or yard work in areas to which cats have access. Serologic testing of domestic cats is not useful.

Neither patients with acquired toxoplasmosis nor neonates with congenital toxoplasmosis require isolation.

The regimen of choice for treating acute toxoplasmosis is either the synergistic combination of pyrimethamine plus sulfadiazine or trisulfapyrimidine. Unfortunately, pyrimethamine is not only potentially toxic but also potentially teratogenic. Limited studies, however, indicate that the frequency of congenital toxoplasmosis is reduced in neonates of pregnant women acutely infected after the first trimester if the women are treated with the combination of drugs; treatment is recommended. Neonates with active congenital disease should also be treated early because therapy may prevent further tissue invasion and destruction. Furthermore, asymptomatic infected neonates should be treated to try to prevent late sequelae.

Chlamydial Infections

Chlamydia trachomatis has been detected in the cervix of approximately 5%–7% of pregnant women; the prevalence varies widely in different population groups. Most infected women are asymptomatic, but *Chlamydia* may cause purulent (nongonococcal) cervicitis. Purulent conjunctivitis occurs in approximately 30%–50% of neonates born vaginally to women infected with *Chlamydia*, and neonatal pneumonia occurs in 10%–20%.

Chlamydial infections in pregnant women may be treated with erythromycin. Chlamydial infections in the neonate are generally mild and responsive to antimicrobial therapy; prophylactic cesarean delivery is not warranted. Prophylactic use of topical erythromycin, and possibly topical tetracycline, instilled into the conjuctival sac of the neonate shortly after birth may prevent inclusion conjunctivitis, but it probably will not prevent chlamydial pneumonia.

Neonates with inclusion conjunctivitis should be managed with drainage/secretion precautions. Those with chlamydial pneumonia should be managed similarly and separated from neonates who are uninfected and neonates who are infected with other respiratory agents. Transmission of chlamydial infections within nurseries has been suspected but not proved.

OTHER INFECTIOUS PROBLEMS DURING PREGNANCY

Antepartum Problems

Pyelonephritis

Most women who develop pyelonephritis during pregnancy enter pregnancy with asymptomatic bacteriuria. Urine should be screened for bacteria in selected patients (e.g., in patients with a history of urinary tract infection or renal disease). Significant bacteriuria, once detected, should be treated appropriately, and follow-up cultures should be done periodically to ensure eradication of infection and to rule out recurrence.

Pregnant patients with overt pyelonephritis may go into premature labor or septic shock. Accordingly, when pyelonephritis is diagnosed in pregnancy, it should be treated vigorously in the hospital with appropriate antibiotics.

Immunization During Pregnancy

Immunizing agents are not usually indicated during pregnancy, although there is no evidence that commonly used, inactivated bacterial or viral vaccines or toxoids have an adverse effect on the mother or fetus. Live virus vaccines should not be given except in the rare case in which the patient has been exposed to yellow fever or polio and the disease poses a greater threat than does vaccination. Pregnancy is a contraindication to vaccination against rubella, measles, and mumps, since these vaccines contain live, attenuated virus. Recommendations for vaccinations during pregnancy are shown in Table 6–2.

Intrapartum Infection (Clinical Chorioamnionitis)

Chorioamnionitis is diagnosed in approximately 1% of all pregnancies; it is diagnosed in a larger percentage of pregnancies with prolonged membrane rupture. Although signs and symptoms are often nonspecific, the infection should be suspected when maternal fever, maternal or fetal tachycardia, foul odor, or uterine tenderness develops. Evaluation of infection in the mother should include a complete blood count, blood culture, and a genital culture. Therapy consists of supportive care, delivery, and antibiotics. The obstetrician should inform the nursery staff of the suspected diagnosis so that the neonate's condition may be evaluated appropriately.

Postpartum Infection

Nursery staff should be informed of any suspected or confirmed maternal disease. Sustained maternal fever may be the sole indicator.

Genital Infection (Endometritis)

Endometritis occurs after 1%–3% of vaginal deliveries and complicates 10%–50% of cesarean deliveries. Genital infections are frequently more severe after cesarean delivery than after vaginal delivery. Risk factors for infection include prolonged labor or membrane rupture, lower socioeconomic status, anemia, and trauma. Most studies have found that internal fetal monitoring does not directly increase infection rates in the mother. Onset of endometritis is usually within the first few days after delivery and is characterized by fever, malaise, tachycardia, abdominal pain, or foul lochia. Localizing signs may be absent early in the course of infection.

The condition of febrile postpartum patients should be evaluated by means of a pertinent history, complete physical examination, blood count, and blood, genital, and urine cultures. Bacteria most likely to cause infection are the gram-negative enteric aerobes (especially *Escherichia coli*), selected aerobic streptococci (α-hemolytic streptococci, group B β-hemolytic streptococci, and the enterococci), gram-negative anaerobic rods (especially *Bacteroides fragilis*), and anaerobic cocci (*Peptococcus* and *Peptostreptococcus*). Infections may be mixed, and anaerobic

Table 6–2. *Recommendations for Active and Passive Immunization During Pregnancy**

Immunizable disease	Vaccine/biologic: Indications for immunization
	Live, Attenuated Virus Vaccines
Poliomyelitis	Avoid vaccine use if possible. Live oral polio vaccine (OPV) recommended only if immediate risk of exposure to wild virus is substantial. Inactivated polio vaccine (IPV) may be used if there is time to complete immunization before exposure.
Measles	Vaccine contraindicated. Passive immunization with immune globulin, 0.25 ml/kg body weight (maximum dose, 15 ml) as soon after exposure as possible may attenuate infection.
Mumps	Vaccine contraindicated during pregnancy.
Rubella	Vaccine contraindicated during pregnancy.
Yellow fever	Vaccine contraindicated except for unavoidable exposure to disease before end of pregnancy.
Smallpox	No current indication.
	Inactivated Virus Vaccines
Hepatitis B	Vaccine not contraindicated during pregnancy in a susceptible woman at high risk of hepatitis B infection. Risk of vaccine to the fetus should be negligible, although data on safety are not available.
Influenza	Standard vaccine recommendations, i.e., high-risk underlying conditions, such as pulmonary, cardiac, or renal disease. If possible, avoid administration during first trimester.
Rabies	Pregnancy does not alter indications for postexposure prophylaxis with rabies immune globulin and vaccine. Preexposure prophylaxis may be indicated if risk of exposure to rabies is substantial.
	Live, Attenuated Bacterial Vaccine
Tuberculosis	BCG vaccine contraindicated during pregnancy unless immediate risk of unavoidable exposure to infective tuberculosis is excessive.
	Inactivated Bacterial Vaccines
Typhoid	Vaccine contraindicated except for close, continued exposure to carrier or travel to endemic areas.
Cholera	Vaccine contraindicated except to meet international travel requirements.
Meningococcal infection	Vaccine safety during pregnancy not established; avoid unless risk of exposure is substantial.
Pneumococcal infection	Vaccine safety during pregnancy not established; avoid unless risk of exposure is substantial.
Plague	No information available on safety of vaccine during pregnancy. Highly selective vaccination of individuals at substantial risk of disease.
	Toxoids
Tetanus, diphtheria	Booster dose of adult TD toxoid (tetanus, full dose; diphtheria, reduced dose) if primary series incomplete or no booster within 10 years. Primary series for unimmunized woman.

*For all products, consult the manufacturer's package insert for instruction for storage, handling, and administration. Biologics prepared by different manufacturers may vary.

genital culture may reveal organisms that require special precautions or special therapy. Isolation procedures appropriate to the suspected type of infection should be instituted promptly.

Patients usually respond promptly to antibiotic therapy, but persistent fever, retained infected placenta, septic pelvic thrombophlebitis, or pelvic abscess are occasional complications.

Mastitis

Infection of the breast usually develops during or after the second week postpartum, most often after the patient has been discharged from the hospital. Local breast inflammation, often with fever, is the predominant sign. The breast secretions should be cultured and antimicrobial susceptibilities determined. Since *S. aureus* is commonly the cause, the antibiotic selected should be active against this organism, as well as others; oral agents such as dicloxacillin or a cephalosporin are reasonable initial choices. Local warm compresses and analgesics are helpful adjunctive measures. Frank abscesses, which occur infrequently, require drainage. Opinions vary about the advisability of continuing breast-feeding. If there is no abscess that requires drainage, feeding from the uninfected breast can usually be continued; the involved breast should be expressed manually or with a breast pump.

Puerperal Sepsis

Although epidemic nosocomial infections on obstetric services may be caused by a number of viral and bacterial pathogens, most epidemics have involved infections with group A streptococci. Epidemics of such lethal infections were reported as late as 1927, and the threat of group A streptococcal infection has remained long after the introduction of penicillin. Since this organism is an unusual inhabitant of the vagina, the source of the epidemic is usually a hospital staff member rather than a patient. After the organism has been introduced into a unit, however, infected patients serve as reservoirs, and infection is transmitted from one patient to another on the hands of personnel.

Epidemics are better prevented than controlled. Specimens taken from sites of probable group A streptococcal infection (e.g., throat or skin) in obstetric personnel should be cultured. Personnel found to have streptococcal infection should be treated with appropriate doses of penicillin or erythromycin for 10 days and prohibited from providing direct patient care until cultures are negative. Patients with group A streptococcal infection should be managed with contact isolation until treatment has been initiated with appropriate doses of penicillin or other antibiotics effective against the organism involved. Hospital personnel must observe hand-washing and isolation recommendations meticulously.

If two or more cases of group A streptococcal infection develop within a short interval, hospital infection control personnel should be notified. In addition to isolation and treatment of infected patients, control may require screening patients and personnel by cultures, and possibly treatment for carriers. Anal and vaginal carrier-disseminators of group A streptococci have been documented. To assist in the epidemiologic evaluation, isolates should be saved and submitted to the state health department laboratory for M and T typing. During severe epidemics, patients should receive prophylactic penicillin or sulfonamide, and it may be necessary to cancel elective surgery and cesarean deliveries.

MANAGEMENT OF NURSERY OUTBREAKS OF DISEASE

Since many infections become apparent only after neonates leave the hospital, each hospital should establish a procedure to be used for disease surveillance of recently discharged neonates during a suspected or confirmed epidemic. Procedures for control of nursery epidemics depend on the microorganism responsible for the outbreak, the reservoir of infection, and the mode of transmission. An epidemiologic investigation should be undertaken to identify these factors. The local hospital infection control committee and the proper health authorities should be notified promptly about all suspected or confirmed epidemics.

During epidemics, a total program of infection control is required. If a problem is suspected, the first step is to evaluate it promptly and carefully. The result of this initial assessment determines the need for further epidemiologic studies to define the source and means of transmission of the infections, as well as the type of specific control measures that are required. Even if an intensive investigation is not indicated, the results of the control measures should be evaluated to ensure that they have been effective and the problem has been resolved.

Surveillance for *Staphylococcus aureus*

Colonization of newborns by *S. aureus* is relatively common, but disease is usually sporadic; frequency of disease is dependent on multiple factors, including the virulence of the colonizing strain. Although the prevalence of *S. aureus* colonization of neonates fluctuates and may at times be over 50%, nurseries with good infection control practices frequently are able to restrict neonate colonization rates to 20% or less. *S. aureus* disease occurs with any prevalence of colonization in the nursery, however. Most frequently, disease caused by infection with *S. aureus* occurs in neonates during the second week of postnatal life, after the neonates have been discharged from the nursery. Infections detected in neonates before discharge from the nursery, therefore, may represent only a small fraction of the total.

Generally, *S. aureus* is transmitted to neonates on the inadequately washed hands of personnel; colonized and infected neonates serve as the reservoir. Rarely, a personnel disseminator, with or without staphylococcal lesions, is responsible for a cluster of infections. Most colonized personnel do not disseminate their organisms, however, and the colonization by this means is epidemiologically insignificant. Fomites are not usually implicated in the transmission of *S. aureus* infections.

A presumptive epidemic in a nursery may be defined as the occurrence of cutaneous infections in two or more neonates simultaneously (or within a short period of time) or the development of a breast abscess in a mother or a deep infection in a neonate. Another rough guideline is that no more than 3–4 full-term neonates per 1000 live births should develop *S. aureus* infection while in the nursery. If an epidemic or unacceptably high frequency of infection is suspected, the following steps should be taken:

1. Determine if an epidemic is probable by preparing a careful log (line-listing) of each neonate with proved or suspected staphylococcal disease, including date of onset, location of the neonate within the nursery, personnel caring for the neonate, and characteristics of the causative organism (antibiotic susceptibility pattern and phage type, if available). Rates of disease should also be calculated for convenient periods of time to establish trends of disease.

2. Determine the degree of asymptomatic colonization of neonates with *S. aureus* by culturing tissue from the umbilical stumps and anterior nares of neonates currently in the involved nursery areas. Isolates of *S. aureus,* as well as all the isolates from neonates with clinical infections, should be saved by the laboratory for phage typing or additional studies. A complete antibiotic susceptibility pattern and, if available, phage typing should be performed on all isolates to determine if disease is caused by a single strain, signaling a possible common source nosocomial problem. Prevalence culture surveys should be conducted regularly during the

outbreak to monitor colonization status of neonates and assess the results of control measures.

3. Determine the extent of disease in neonates recently discharged from the hospital, either by a survey of physicians or providers taking care of most neonates born in the hospital or by a telephone survey of parents of the neonates. Health departments or nursing associations may provide assistance with the survey.

4. If the disease is mild and the disease rate is low, reemphasize meticulous patient care techniques, and institute cohorts for infected and colonized neonates and for all new admissions to the nursery units. A strictly enforced cohort system for both neonates and personnel virtually eliminates contact between infected and unexposed neonates, interrupting disease transmission. Careful handwashing by all personnel after each contact with a neonate is particularly important. This approach may decrease colonization and control the problem. Some epidemics have been controlled by treatment of the cord and the nose with an antibiotic ointment (such as bacitracin ointment) or by treatment of the cord with triple dye.

5. Examine personnel for the presence of cutaneous lesions, especially on the hands, that may be caused by *S. aureus*. Material from lesions should be cultured, and the individual should be removed from patient care activities in the nursery until the lesions have healed. If the outbreak is caused by a single strain of *S. aureus* and cannot be controlled promptly, an epidemiologic investigation should be conducted to search for a carrier-disseminator among the personnel. It may be necessary to culture the anterior nares of personnel to detect carriers of the epidemic strain; phage typing should also be done on these isolates. Personnel carrying the epidemic strain are usually inadvertently colonized and are not epidemiologic disseminators. They should be treated intranasally with topical antibiotics (e.g., bacitracin); cultures should be done after treatment has been completed. Personnel colonized with the epidemic strain may continue to provide care for neonates already colonized or infected. Any individual identified epidemiologically as a disseminator, however, should be removed from patient care responsibilities pending successful eradication of colonization. Persistent disseminators may need more vigorous treatment or special evaluation or therapy. Expert consultation may be necessary.

6. Continue surveillance in the nursery for several weeks after the epidemic has apparently terminated. Observation for disease in

neonates (both in the nursery and at home for several weeks after discharge) is the most reliable index. Weekly cultures from neonates (umbilical cord and nares) in the nursery and from nares of personnel may be valuable for a short time, but they are not useful routinely. Long periods of serial surveillance of neonates and personnel are not practical. Monitoring of neonates for *S. aureus* is probably the best method for determining the need for prevalence surveys in neonates or personnel.

Until the outbreak is under control, full-term neonates who weigh at least 2500 g should have the diaper area only bathed with a preparation containing 3% hexachlorophene as soon after birth as possible and daily until they are discharged. Hexachlorophene must be used with caution because systemic absorption with central nervous system damage has been reported. It should not be used as a routine, and it must not be used for preterm or low-birth-weight neonates.

In serious outbreaks, or if the foregoing procedures are not effective, bacterial interference or administration of a systemic antibiotic to all neonates may be justified; expert consultation should be obtained before resorting to these measures, however.

Infectious Diarrhea: *Escherichia coli*

Measures for management of a nursery epidemic of diarrheal disease caused by *E. coli* are also appropriate for management of diarrheal disease caused by other bacterial (e.g., *Salmonella*) or viral pathogens. The reservoir of infection is usually the intestinal tract of ill or colonized neonates and infection is usually transmitted from neonate to neonate on the inadequately washed hands of personnel. Occasionally, other sources, such as extrinsically contaminated formula, may be found.

The epidemic strain of *E. coli* should be determined. Epidemic enteric disease may be caused by (1) strains of enterotoxin-producing *E. coli* that may or may not be agglutinated by commercial antisera or (2) specific enteropathogenic *E. coli* that do not usually produce known enterotoxins. When a single strain of *E. coli* (identified by colony characteristics and antimicrobial susceptibility pattern) is isolated from a large number of symptomatic neonates and can be associated with the outbreak (i.e., the strain is predominant or pure in cultures from ill neonates, it is isolated from them much more often than from those who remain well, and no other obvious pathogen such as *Shigella* or *Salmonella* is present), it should be serotyped and tested for enterotoxin production if this can be done quickly and reliably by available laboratories.

Because asymptomatic carriage of an identifiable pathogen may perpetuate an outbreak, a rectal specimen for culture should be obtained from all neonates in proximity to the index case or other symptomatic neonates. Fluorescent antibody studies, if available, may help identify the pathogen within hours.

Diseased and colonized neonates must be placed into strict cohort and segregated from the other neonates; personnel providing care for the culture-positive neonates should not provide care for neonates who have not been infected or colonized. Reduction in the number of neonates in the nursery is helpful. In some outbreaks it may be necessary to close the nursery to all new admissions and to make other arrangements.

Appropriate antibiotics should be administered to all neonates excreting the epidemic strain. If serotype information is not available to identify the epidemic strain, all symptomatic neonates, as well as those in the same room or cohort, should be treated. Antibiotic selection must be based on susceptibility tests. Colistin (10–15 mg/kg/day) or neomycin (100 mg/kg/day), administered orally in three or four doses for 5 days, may be useful. Although this duration of treatment may be adequate, neonates who must remain in the nursery should be treated until their stools no longer contain the pathogenic strain (as determined by fluorescent antibody study or culture of three consecutive specimens obtained after completion of antibiotic therapy). During an outbreak, prophylactic administration of colistin or neomycin to all neonates may be appropriate, although efficacy may be variable.

Personnel who are carriers of the epidemic organism have been implicated only rarely as the source of an epidemic, but they should be identified by culture of stool specimens. Carrier-disseminators should be removed from the nursery until they have been treated and are culture-negative.

Antiseptic and aseptic techniques should be reviewed and strictly observed. Particular emphasis should be placed on hand-washing by personnel between neonate contacts. Requiring personnel to use gowns when in contact with diseased or colonized neonates and to wash their hands, even after using disposable gloves, when handling infected neonates and contaminated materials may reduce the degree of contamination of hands and clothing by the infecting pathogen.

Although transmission by contaminated fomites is uncommon, nursery practices should be evaluated; equipment that may be contaminated, especially solutions or articles that would have contact with the gastrointestinal tract of neonates, may need to be cultured. After all infected or colonized neonates have been discharged, the nursery, including equipment, should be thoroughly cleaned and disinfected. Neonates recently discharged should be surveyed. All symptomatic neonates should be examined, specimens obtained for culture, and treatment provided. Surveillance by periodic examination of cultures from neonates, personnel, and other sources of contamination should be continued for a short period after the outbreak has been controlled. If the pathogen is not recovered from cultures, surveillance can be stopped.

Klebsiella and Other Gram-Negative Bacteria

Gram-negative bacteria, especially *Klebsiella pneumoniae*, frequently cause infections in nurseries, particularly in intensive care nurseries. Strains of these bacteria resistant to multiple antibiotics, including gentamicin, kanamycin, and chloramphenicol, are becoming increasingly common. These organisms may be virulent, invasive, and unusually difficult to eradicate.

Infection control procedures should be instituted promptly if organisms with these characteristics are identified in the unit. Although clinical infection may occur at various sites, the intestinal tract is the most frequent site of colonization; therefore, stool cultures (and perhaps cultures from other sites) should be obtained from all neonates in the nursery to identify rapidly those who are colonized. Selective media containing antibiotics may be used to simplify isolating the specific pathogen.

The infected neonates should be segregated and managed with appropriate isolation precautions (e.g., contact isolation or enteric precautions). Neonate isolation techniques should include the use of disposable diapers and gloves. A strict cohort system should be established immediately. Personnel providing care for infected or colonized neonates should not provide care for uninfected neonates as transmission appears to occur despite careful hand-washing.

The pattern of antibiotic use in the nursery may have to be altered periodically to avoid resistance.

Necrotizing Enterocolitis

Neonates in the nursery may develop necrotizing enterocolitis, an illness defined pathologically or by pneumatosis intestinalis on an abdominal radiograph and a symptom complex including abdominal distention, gastrointestinal bleeding, gastric retention, and palpable loops of bowel. Necrotizing enterocolitis occurs predominantly in preterm neonates; although neonates at high risk of disease can be identified, the etiology and pathophysiology are poorly understood. The organisms frequently associated with the disorder include *K. pneumoniae, E. coli,* and *Clostridium difficile.* Cases often occur in clusters, and several investigators have noted that neonates with bowel colonization with specific strains of bacteria are more likely to develop necrotizing enterocolitis than neonates colonized with different strains.

These data suggest that it may be prudent to manage neonates with suspected or confirmed necrotizing enterocolitis with enteric precautions, including gown and gloves when working directly with the neonate or articles likely to be contaminated with feces. A cluster of cases may require establishing a strict cohort of neonates colonized with a common bacterial strain. A cohort of personnel caring for the affected neonates also should be established.

Administration of prophylactic oral or systemic antibiotics in an effort to prevent necrotizing enterocolitis in neonates has not been successful and is likely to result in the emergence of resistant bacteria.

Group A β-Hemolytic *Streptococcus*

Epidemics of infection with strains of group A β-hemolytic streptococci are uncommon at present. If this problem arises, the following steps are recommended:

1. Determine the extent of the epidemic by culturing any lesions and the umbilical stumps of all neonates in the nursery.

2. Institute a cohort system. The nursery need not be closed to new admissions.

3. Employ the various approaches that have been used to control epidemics, including isolation and treatment of all culture-positive neonates, fomite control, and careful hand-washing. In all instances, a complete epidemiologic investigation with isolation or treatment of carriers is essential to successful control. Use isolation techniques (e.g., drainage/secretion precautions, physical segregation) for all neonates who have had contact with infected persons to reduce the number of colonized neonates in the nursery who may serve as a reservoir for infection.

4. Provide prophylaxis for all neonates with benzathine penicillin G (50,000 units/kg body weight); treat neonates with disease caused by group A streptococci with penicillin G (50,000–100,000 units/ kg body weight/day in two or three divided doses) for 5–10 days.

5. Conduct a telephone survey of the parents or pediatricians of recently discharged, exposed neonates to determine whether any neonate is ill, although most neonates carrying group A *Streptococcus* will be free of disease or will have only a mild omphalitis. Examine symptomatic neonates and obtain specimens for culture; institute antibiotic treatment, if appropriate.

6. Obtain culture specimens from the nose, throat, and any cutaneous lesion of all nursery personnel. Anal carriage of group A streptococci has been implicated as the cause of epidemics of surgical wound infections; to avoid the need for anal cultures from all personnel, epidemiologic techniques should be used, if necessary, to try to determine those few personnel most likely to be disseminating infection. Personnel with positive cultures should be removed from the nursery and treated until cultures are negative.

7. Continue surveillance in the nursery for several weeks after the epidemic has ended. Obtain specimens for culture from neonates just before they are discharged. If the problem persists, weekly nose and throat cultures of nursery personnel may be indicated.

THE ENVIRONMENT: CLEANING, DISINFECTION, AND STERILIZATION

The physician in charge and the nursing supervisor of the obstetric and nursery areas should work with the infection control officer and other groups as appropriate (e.g., representatives of the respiratory therapy service, central supply, and housekeeping) to establish an environmental control program for the labor, delivery, and nursery areas. This program should include specific procedures in a written policy manual for cleaning and disinfection or sterilization of patient care areas, equipment, and supplies. Consultation for specific details and problems is essential. Nursing supervisors should ensure that these procedures are carried out correctly.

Methods of Sterilizing and Disinfecting Patient Care Equipment

All medical and hospital personnel should understand the difference between sterilization and disinfection. Sterilization is the destruction of all microorganisms, including spores; disinfection is simply a reduction in the number of contaminating microorganisms. High-level disinfection is the elimination or destruction of all microorganisms except spores. Cleaning is the physical removal of organic material or soil, including microorganisms from objects. Equipment that enters normally sterile tissue or the vascular system must be sterile. For neonates, equipment that comes into contact with mucous membranes or that has prolonged or intimate contact with skin should also be sterile. Much of the equipment required in perinatal care areas can be used safely if it is satisfactorily cleaned and disinfected; clean, dry surfaces do not support the growth of microorganisms.

It is sometimes necessary to decontaminate equipment before it is sterilized or disinfected in order to allow processing without the risk of exposure to hazardous microbes. Then the equipment must be cleaned thoroughly to remove all blood, tissue, secretions, food, and other residue. Without thorough cleaning, no method of sterilization or disinfection can be effective. In addition, some chemical disinfectants are inactivated by organic materials.

Sterilization

Methods of sterilization include steam (autoclaving), dry heat and gaseous (ethylene oxide) or liquid chemical (e.g., 2% glutaraldehyde) techniques. The preferred method of sterilization is steam autoclaving, because this is the least expensive method and provides the greatest margin of safety. Some equipment may be damaged by steam, however, and must be sterilized by another method.

Equipment sterilized with ethylene oxide usually requires 8–12 hours of aeration before it can be used again if the equipment material absorbs ethylene oxide. Ethylene oxide sterilization of supplies or equipment should be preceded by a comprehensive review of authoritative data on the aeration time required for each material to be processed and the extent to which toxicity standards have been established. An ethylene oxide sterilization plan also requires availability of sufficient equipment to allow time for aeration.

Equipment that cannot be sterilized with steam or ethylene oxide may be satisfactorily sterilized after cleaning by immersion for 10 hours in 2% glutaraldehyde or other acceptable liquid sporicide; this should be followed by three rinses with sterile water (or tap water with at least 10 mg/liter hypochlorite), thorough drying, and packaging in sterile wrappers.

High-Level Disinfection

Equipment that does not need to be sterilized may be subjected to high-level disinfection. Both hot water pasteurization and chemical disinfection are satisfactory. Pasteurization of equipment requires immersing it in water at 80°–85° C (176°–185° F) for 15 minutes or 75° C (167° F) for 30 minutes. After air drying (preferably in a cabinet with heated, filtered air), disinfected items should be aseptically wrapped and stored until needed. Although spores are not eradicated by this method, bacterial decontamination is adequate. The original reports of the equipment manufacturer should be consulted for a list of any parts or materials that may be warped or damaged at these temperatures.

The choice of liquid chemicals for high-level disinfection depends on the type of equipment to be disinfected. In many instances, immersion of the equipment for 30 minutes in 2% glutaraldehyde or an iodophor solution (500 ppm available iodine), followed by three rinses with sterile water (or tap water with at least 10 mg/liter hypochlorite) and thorough drying, is satisfactory.

Cleaning and Disinfecting Noncritical Surfaces

Selection of Disinfectants

Although numerous disinfectants are available, no single agent or preparation is ideal for all purposes. Consideration should be given to the agent and its special use and to the types of organisms likely to be contaminating the object that is to be disinfected. Special attention should be given to the recommended concentration of each disinfectant and its time of exposure. Unnecessary exposure of neonates to disinfectants should be avoided, and strict adherence to manufacturers' recommendations is essential.

Hexachlorophene preparations are not disinfectants and should not be used on equipment or environmental surfaces. Iodophors, chlorine compounds, phenolic compounds, and glutaraldehyde are satisfactory disinfectants. Only iodophor or quaternary disinfectant-detergent products registered by the U.S. Environmental Protection Agency and recommended by the manufacturer as suitable for nursery surfaces with which neonates have contact should be used. Phenolic compounds, especially if used in inappropriate concentrations or on surfaces with which neonates have direct contact, have been associated in exposed infants with hyperbilirubinemia.

General Housekeeping

The following order of cleaning is recommended:

1. Patient areas

2. Accessory areas
3. Adjacent halls

It is not known if floor bacteria are a source of nosocomial infection, but regular cleaning prevents reservoirs of pathogenic bacteria from accumulating. Disinfectant-detergents have been shown to be more effective than soap and water alone in cleaning floors, although hospital floors are rapidly recontaminated after disinfection. Available disinfectant-detergents may differ in effectiveness.

In the cleaning procedure, dust should not be dispersed into the air. Removal of dust by a dry vacuum machine, followed by a wet vacuum pick-up machine, is effective in cleaning and disinfecting hospital floors. Once dust has been removed, scrubbing with a mop and disinfectant-detergent solution should be sufficient. Mop heads should be machine-laundered and thoroughly dried daily.

Standard types of portable vacuum cleaners should not be used in nurseries or delivery areas because particulate matter and microbial contamination in the room may be disturbed and distributed by the exhaust jet. Vacuum cleaners that discharge outside the nursery, i.e., central vacuum cleaning systems or portable vacuums used so that only the cleaning wand, floor tool, and vacuum hose are brought into the nursery, should be used. Central vacuum cleaning systems are most efficiently installed during extensive remodeling or construction of new units.

Cabinet counters, work surfaces, and similar horizontal areas may be subject to heavy contamination during routine use. These areas should be cleaned at least once a day with a disinfectant-detergent and clean cloths; friction cleaning is important to ensure physical removal of dirt and contaminating microorganisms. Surfaces that are contaminated by patient specimens or accidental spills should be carefully cleaned and disinfected; iodophors formulated for environmental cleaning, phenolic compounds, or hypochlorite are useful disinfectants for this type of surface decontamination.

Walls, windows, and storage shelves may be reservoirs of pathogenic microorganisms if grossly soiled or if dust and dirt are allowed to accumulate. These areas—particularly windowsills and other horizontal surfaces—and similar noncritical surfaces should be scrubbed periodically with a disinfectant-detergent solution as part of the general housekeeping program. Aerosols of phenolic or other disinfectants are not reliable for disinfecting hard surfaces; this method is not recommended.

Faucet aerators may be useful to reduce water splashing in sinks;

however, aerators are notoriously susceptible to contamination with a variety of water-loving bacteria. If aerators are used, removing them periodically for cleaning and disinfection or sterilization should reduce contamination, at least temporarily. Sinks and drain traps are usually heavily contaminated, frequently with the same bacteria causing infections in patients; epidemiologically, however, these bacterial reservoirs have only rarely been implicated as the source of the bacteria infecting neonates. Sinks should be scrubbed clean daily with a disinfectant-detergent; drain traps should not need routine cleaning or disinfection.

Written policies should be established for the removal and disposal of solid wastes. Sturdy plastic liners should be used in trash receptacles; these liners should be sealed before being removed from the trash receptacles. In patient care areas trash receptacles should be cleaned and disinfected regularly. Infectious material requires special handling and disposal.

Special housekeeping personnel should be assigned to clean the nursery. If the nursery is small, they also may be assigned to work in the obstetric areas or other "clean" areas of the hospital, e.g., offices, psychiatric services, or elective surgical areas. Housekeeping personnel assigned permanently to the obstetric or nursery areas should wear scrub uniforms as do other full-time personnel; those not assigned to these areas exclusively should wear clean gowns when entering the areas. Daily cleaning of the nursery should take place when most neonates are not present.

Cleaning and Disinfecting Patient Care Equipment

Incubators and Bassinets

After a neonate has been discharged, the incubator or bassinet used by that neonate should be cleaned and disinfected thoroughly. An iodophor or quaternary ammonium disinfectant-detergent registered by the U.S. Environmental Protection Agency is recommended for this purpose. Manufacturers' directions should be followed carefully. A bassinet or incubator should never be cleaned when occupied. Infants who remain in the nursery for an extended period should be transferred to a cleaned and disinfected isolette periodically.

When an incubator is being cleaned and disinfected, all detachable parts should be removed and scrubbed meticulously. If the ventilation unit has a fan, it should be cleaned carefully and disinfected; manufacturer's instructions should be followed to avoid equipment damage. The air filter need not be discarded each time the incubator is cleaned, but it should be removed and autoclaved weekly or each time the unit is cleaned. Mattresses should be replaced when the surface covering is broken, because this precludes effective disinfection or sterilization. Mattresses may be sterilized by heat or gas. Portholes and porthole cuffs and sleeves are easily contaminated, often heavily; cuffs should be replaced on a regular schedule or cleaned and disinfected frequently with freshly prepared mild soap or quaternary ammonium disinfectant-detergent solutions. Incubators not in use should be thoroughly dried by running the incubator "hot" without water in the reservoir for 24 hours after disinfection.

Evaporative humidifiers in incubators usually do not produce contaminated aerosols, but contaminated water reservoirs may be responsible for direct rather than airborne transmission of infection. Reservoirs should be filled only with sterile water; they should be drained and refilled with sterile water every 24 hours. Environmental humidity in many areas of the United States or in hospitals with a central ventilation system may be sufficiently high that additional humidification is unnecessary for most neonates and water reservoirs may be left dry. If humidification is necessary, a source of humidity external to the incubator that can be changed daily and sent for cleaning and sterilization or disinfection may be preferable to incubator humidifiers.

Nebulizers and Water Traps

Nebulizers are easily contaminated. Therefore, nebulizers and attached tubing should be replaced by clean, sterile equipment (or equipment that has been subjected to high-level disinfection) every 12–24 hours. Failure to replace tubing may result in contamination of freshly cleaned equipment. Water traps should also be replaced daily by autoclaved or disinfected equipment. Only sterile water should be used for nebulizers or water traps; residual water should be discarded when these containers are refilled. Water condensed in tubing loops should be removed and discarded and should not be allowed to reflux into the container.

Other Equipment

Cleaning and disinfection or sterilization of equipment should be performed between uses on successive patients. Equipment that is used for only one patient should be replaced and cleaned and disinfected or sterilized according to an established schedule. For many types of equipment, this may be at least once a day. Disposable equipment should be replaced with approximately the same frequency as reusable equipment is recycled. Disposable equipment must never be reused.

Resuscitators, face masks, and other items used in direct contact with neonates should be dismantled, thoroughly cleaned, and sterilized, if possible. Alternatively, the equipment may be subjected to high-level disinfection with liquid chemicals or by pasteurization. Equipment such as tubing for respiratory or oxygen therapy should be either sterilized or disposed of after use.

Stethoscopes and similar types of diagnostic instruments should be wiped with an iodophor or alcohol before use. Tubing, connectors, and jars of suction machines should be replaced daily with cleaned and sterilized equipment.

Procedures should be established so that the neonate warmers used for resuscitation in the delivery areas are cleaned regularly, as well as after each use; they should always be stocked with clean, sterile equipment and supplies, available and ready for use when needed.

Cultures of Environmental Surfaces and Equipment

Routine cultures of equipment after cleaning and disinfection are expensive and time-consuming; they should not be a substitute for specific, clearly written, and carefully followed procedures for cleaning and disinfection. Cultures of environmental surfaces and equipment may be useful as part of epidemiologic investigations, however, and an occasional, selective bacteriologic survey of particular patient care areas or equipment may help determine the effectiveness of existing procedures. These studies should be coordinated with the infection control committee and the microbiology laboratory.

Neonatal Linen

Procedures for laundering, making up packs, and delivering linen to the nursery should be established by the medical, nursing, laundry, and administrative staffs of the hospital.

Each delivery of clean linen should contain sufficient linen for at least one 8-hour shift. Linen should be brought to the nursery from the laundry in a closed cabinet that can also serve as the storage unit. If this system is not used, the linen should be stored in specifically designated cabinets in a clean area of the laundry. Traditionally, linen used in the intensive care, intermediate care, continuing care, and admission/observation areas is autoclaved, but the need for this to prevent infections in newborns has not been established by any studies. Autoclaved linen is probably not necessary in normal newborn care areas.

No new garments or linen should be used for neonates without prior laundering. To prevent methemoglobinemia, garments should not be marked with aniline dyes.

Disposable Diapers

Not only are disposable diapers acceptable alternatives to cloth diapers in a nursery, but those that have been sterilized by the manufacturer are preferred for small neonates, those with diaper rash, and those with other skin lesions that are prone to secondary infection. Disposable diapers not labeled as sterile may be acceptable for other neonates. The importance of nonsterile diapers in the epidemiology of neonatal disease has not been established.

Care of Soiled Linen

An established procedure for disposal of soiled linen should be strictly followed. Chutes for the transfer of soiled linen from patient care areas to the laundry are not acceptable unless they are under negative air pressure. Soiled linen should be discarded into impervious plastic bags placed in hampers that are easy to clean and disinfect. Soiled diapers should be placed into special diaper receptacles immediately after removal from the neonate; they should never be rinsed in the nursery. All personnel should be aware that handling dirty diapers with bare hands can result in heavy contamination and transient colonization of the hands with microorganisms that cannot be eliminated easily with hand-washing and can be readily transmitted to the next neonate for whom care is provided.

Plastic bags of soiled diapers (reusable or disposable) and other linen should be sealed and removed from the nursery at least every 8 hours. Individuals who collect the bags of soiled diapers or linen need not enter the nursery if all bags are placed outside the nursery. Sealed bags of reusable, soiled nursery linens should be taken to the laundry at least twice each day; sealed bags of disposable diapers also should be taken away at least twice a day.

Laundering

Diapers and soiled linen should not be removed from their sealed bags until they reach the laundry. They should be washed separately from other hospital linen. It is important that nursery linen remain soft. The souring operation, which neutralizes the alkalis used in the washing process and is responsible for the greatest bacterial destruction, is appropriate.

Fatal pentachlorophenol poisoning has been observed when an

antimildew agent containing a high concentration of the sodium salt of this compound was used in the final rinse in a laundry. The chemical trichlorcarbanilide should not be used in hospital laundering because of potential hazard to neonates.

To avoid potential hazards associated with chemicals or enzymes used in the hospital laundry, the physician in charge should know of all agents in use and should be informed before any changes are made in the chemicals or laundry procedures used. Currently, there are no legal requirements for testing laundry or cleaning agents for special hazards to neonates. Therefore, caution must be exercised when new agents are introduced to the nursery or when laundry or cleaning procedures are changed.

RESOURCES AND RECOMMENDED READING

American Academy of Pediatrics: Report of the Committee on Infectious Diseases, 19 ed. Evanston, IL, AAP, 1982

American Academy of Pediatrics, Committees on Fetus and Newborn and Infectious Diseases; American College of Obstetricians and Gynecologists, Committee on Obstetrics: Maternal/Fetal Medicine: Perinatal herpes simplex virus infections. Pediatrics 66:147–149, 1980

American College of Obstetricians and Gynecologists: Immunization During Pregnancy (ACOG Technical Bulletin 64). Washington, DC, ACOG, 1982

American College of Surgeons: Manual on Control of Infection in Surgical Patients. Philadelphia, JB Lippincott, 1976

Bennett JV, Brachman PS (eds): Hospital Infections. Boston, Little, Brown, 1979

Centers for Disease Control: Guidelines for the Prevention and Control of Nosocomial Infections. Washington, DC, US Government Printing Office, 1981

Centers for Disease Control: Guideline for Isolation Precautions, 4 ed. Washington, DC, US Government Printing Office, 1983

Feigin RD, Cherry JD (eds): Textbook of Pediatric Infectious Diseases. Philadelphia, WB Saunders, 1981

Remington JS, Klein JO (eds): Infectious Diseases of the Fetus and Newborn Infant. Philadelphia, WB Saunders, 1976

Wenzel RP (ed): Handbook of Hospital Acquired Infections. Boca Raton, FL, CRC Press, 1981 *chapter*

7

Maternal and Newborn Nutrition

Appropriate nutrition is an essential component of the total care of the pregnant woman. Although it is best if a woman develops good eating habits before she becomes pregnant, the physician or other members of the health care team often need to educate the patient who is already pregnant about nutrition. All individuals tend to follow the nutritional habits established during their childhood. However, the months of pregnancy and early puerperium present an opportunity to initiate corrective activities that may improve the quality of life for a woman and her unborn child. Obstetric care usually provides 7–9 months of observation with 15–18 office, clinic, or hospital visits. During these occasions, the health professional may be influential in correcting any inappropriate health habits.

Consultation with a registered dietitian/nutritionist affiliated with a local agency or hospital may be necessary when therapeutic dietary counseling is needed. In addition, pamphlets, many of which contain sample diets, are available from numerous sources, including the American College of Obstetricians and Gynecologists, the Public Health Service, and the March of Dimes–Birth Defects Foundation. If a patient is financially unable to meet her nutritional needs, she should be referred to a social service agency, public assistance program, or the Women, Infants, and Children (WIC) program.

NUTRITION HISTORY

When taking the general medical history, the physician should pay careful attention to the patient's food intake. Factors associated with poor nutrition, such as adolescence, dietary abuse, drug abuse, chronic illness, and abnormal weight, should be noted. Excessive use of alcohol, smoking, or caffeine also affect nutrition by interfering with regular caloric intake.

Pregnancies complicated by hypertension, diabetes, or renal disease require special nutritional management. Counseling may be necessary to ensure that the patient's nutritional needs for pregnancy, as well as for the chronic disease, are met. If possible, the internist, the obstetrician, and a registered dietitian/nutritionist should share therapeutic responsibility.

A history of allergies or food intolerance is also important. Better patient cooperation can be obtained if appropriate substitutes are found for foods that the patient tolerates poorly.

The 24-hour recall is one measure of nutritional intake. The patient should maintain a record of food consumption to measure eating habits. Information that should be noted includes factors such as the timing of meals, emphasis on one type of food, ethnic factors, and intake of items that put the patient at risk.

Table 7–1 lists food requirements for pregnant and lactating women. Vegetarians who include dairy products in their diet usually do not have difficulty meeting nutritional needs during pregnancy. Vegetarians with more restrictive diets may require supplementary iron, folic acid, zinc, and possibly vitamin B_{12}, and they should be referred to a registered dietitian/nutritionist knowledgeable in this area. Adolescents often require nutritional counseling during pregnancy as well.

Table 7–1. *Food Guide for Pregnancy and Lactation*

	Number of servings		
Food groups	Pregnant	Lactating	Pregnant vegetarian (lacto)
Protein foods			
Animal (meat/poultry/fish/eggs)	2	2	—
Legumes/nuts	2	2	3
Milk and milk products	4	5	6
Fruits and vegetables			
Vitamin C rich	1	1	1
Dark green	1	1	1
Other	2	2	3
Whole grain cereal products	4	4	5
Fats and oils	2 tbs	2tbs	2tbs

(California Department of Health: Nutrition During Pregnancy and Lactation, 1977)

During the prenatal physical examination, attention should be paid to the condition of the skin, nails, hair, mouth, teeth, and musculoskeletal system.

WEIGHT GAIN

Mean weight and height values as well as energy needs are shown in Table 7–2. Low prepregnancy weight is defined as 10–15% or more under ideal body weight for height; obesity is defined as 20% over the ideal body weight for height.

The pregnant woman of average weight requires about 2400

Table 7–2. *Mean Heights and Weights and Recommended Energy Intake (Recommended Dietary Allowances Revised 1980)**

Category	Age (yr)	Weight (kg)	Weight (lb)	Height (cm)	Height (in)	Energy needs (with range) (kcal)	Energy needs (with range) (MJ)
Infants	0.0–0.5	6	13	60	24	kg × 115 (95–145)	kg × .48
	0.5–1.0	9	20	71	28	kg × 105 (80–135)	kg × .44
Children	1–3	13	29	90	35	1300 (900–1800)	5.5
	4–6	20	44	112	44	1700 (1800–2300)	7.1
	7–10	28	62	132	52	2400 (1650–3300)	10.1
Males	11–14	45	99	157	62	2700 (2000–3700)	11.3
	15–18	66	145	176	69	2800 (2100–3900)	11.8
	19–22	70	154	177	70	2900 (2500–3300)	12.2
	23–50	70	154	178	70	2700 (2300–3100)	11.3
	51–75	70	154	178	70	2400 (2000–2800)	10.1
	76+	70	154	178	70	2050 (1650–2450)	8.6
Females	11–14	46	101	157	62	2200 (1500–3000)	9.2
	15–18	55	120	163	64	2100 (1200–3000)	8.8
	19–22	55	120	163	64	2100 (1700–2500)	8.8
	23–50	55	120	163	64	2000 (1600–2400)	8.4
	51–75	55	120	163	64	1800 (1400–2200)	7.6
	76+	55	120	163	64	1600 (1200–2000)	6.7
Pregnancy						+300	

*The energy allowances for the young adults are for men and women doing light work. The allowances for the two older groups represent mean energy needs over these age spans, allowing for a 2% decrease in basal (resting) metabolic rate per decade and a reduction in activity of 200 kcal/day for men and women between 51 and 75 years, 500 kcal for men over 75 years and 400 kcal for women over 75. The customary range of daily energy output for adults is shown in parentheses, and is based on a variation in energy needs of ± 400 kcal at any one age, emphasizing the wide range of energy intakes appropriate for any group of people.

Energy allowances for children through age 18 are based on median energy intakes of children of these ages followed in longitudinal growth studies. The values in parentheses are 10th and 90th percentiles of energy intake to indicate the range of energy consumption among children of these ages.

(Food and Nutrition Board, National Academy of Sciences–National Research Council, Washington, DC)

Kcal/day or 36–38 Kcal/kg daily during pregnancy. Most normal weight patients acquire sufficient calories and gain adequate weight by eating to appetite. Inadequate weight gain may be associated with an increased risk of fetal difficulties in utero and low-birth-weight neonates who have problems in the intrapartum and postpartum periods. Inadequate weight gain seems to have its greatest effect in women who are of low or normal weight prior to pregnancy.

Universal agreement has never been achieved on how much weight should be gained during pregnancy. More important than total weight gain is the pattern of weight gain. Maximal gain occurs during the second trimester, although from a practical point of view the rate of gain is essentially linear after the tenth gestational week, averaging about 0.4 kg/week. The usual average total weight gain, therefore, is 10–12 kg (22–27 lb). A graph should be included in the prenatal chart so that weight can be plotted at each visit.

If there has not been a 4–5-kg weight gain by the midpoint of pregnancy, the patient's diet should be reevaluated carefully, and referral to a registered dietitian/nutritionist is essential. The woman who begins prenatal care in the third trimester cannot be expected to compensate for any weight problems to this point. For instance, the patient who gains 9 kg in the first 3 months should not limit her intake and gain only 2.5 kg for the rest of the pregnancy.

All patients, especially those who are obese, should be reminded that they should not begin a weight reduction diet during pregnancy or lactation. In limiting caloric intake, the patient may consume an insufficient amount of essential nutrients, prevent the full utilization of protein, and cause catabolism of fat stores, leading to ketosis and acetonuria.

SPECIFIC NUTRITIONAL NEEDS

The nutritional needs of infants, children, males, females, pregnant women, and lactating mothers are shown in Table 7–3. In all instances, pregnancy and lactation require additional amounts of nutrients for the maintenance of good health.

Iron

Even in the presence of normal hemoglobin and hematocrit levels, the iron stores of many nonpregnant women are depleted because of blood loss during their menstrual periods. During pregnancy, iron stores may be depleted even further. Supplemental iron is needed for both the fetus and the expanded maternal blood volume. The fetus maintains normal hemoglobin and hematocrit levels at the mother's expense, if necessary. This may leave her severely anemic with a decreased oxygen-carrying capacity, increased need for transfusion, and increased susceptibility to infection.

Since the average diet may not adequately meet pregnancy needs, 30–60 mg elemental iron should be given daily to supplement the diet. Iron is found in liver, red meats, dried beans, green leafy vegetables, whole grain enriched bread and cereal, and dried fruits. Iron is more readily absorbed from meat products than from vegetables or grain.

Folic Acid

Since folic acid is required in the formation of heme, the iron-containing protein of hemoglobin, deficiencies in folic acid can affect red cell formation and cause megaloblastic anemia. The folic acid requirement doubles to approximately 800 μg during pregnancy. Folic acid can be found in many of the foods that provide iron and protein. Unless the diet is exceptionally good, however, supplementation with folate is usually required. Supplementation in amounts of a minimum of 400 μg/day is appropriate.

Protein

Cell growth requires protein. Data from studies in laboratory animals suggest that inadequate intake during pregnancy can lead to suboptimal growth of the fetus, decrease the size of various fetal organs, and increase perinatal morbidity and mortality. Nitrogen from protein is present in significant amounts at term in the following tissues: fetus, 55.9 mg; mature placenta, 17 g; amniotic fluid, 1 g; breast tissue, 17g; uterine tissue, 40 g. Most mothers store an additional 200–350 g protein in preparation for losses that occur during labor and parturition, as well as for the physiological demands of lactation. Protein requirements in pregnancy should be calculated on the basis of the patient's maturity and weight. An adult woman needs about 1.3 g protein per day per kilogram of body weight (for an average of about 75 g/day). An adolescent aged 15–18 needs 1.5 g/kg; a younger girl, 1.7 g/kg. About two-thirds of the total protein intake should be of high biologic quality, such as that found in eggs, milk, or meat.

Table 7–3. Recommended Daily Dietary Allowances (Revised 1980)*

	Infants		Children			Males					Females					Pregnant	Lactating
Age (yr)	0.0-0.5	0.5-1.0	1-3	4-6	7-10	11-14	15-18	19-22	23-50	51+	11-14	15-18	19-22	23-50	51+		
Weight																	
kg	6	9	13	20	28	45	66	70	70	70	46	55	55	55	55		
lbs	13	20	29	44	62	99	145	154	154	154	101	120	120	120	120		
Height																	
cm	60	71	90	112	132	157	176	177	178	178	157	163	163	163	163		
in	24	28	35	44	52	62	69	70	70	70	62	64	64	64	64		
Protein (g)	kg×2.2	kg×2.0	23	30	34	45	56	56	56	56	46	46	44	44	44	+30	+20
Fat-Soluble Vitamins																	
Vitamin A (μg R.E.)†	420	400	400	500	700	1000	1000	1000	1000	1000	800	800	800	800	800	+200	+400
Vitamin D (μg)‡	10	10	10	10	10	10	10	7.5	5	5	10	10	7.5	5	5	+5	+5
Vitamin E (mg α T.E.)§	3	4	5	6	7	8	10	10	10	10	8	8	8	8	8	+2	+3
Water-Soluble Vitamins																	
Vitamin C (mg)	35	35	45	45	45	50	60	60	60	60	50	60	60	60	60	+20	+40
Thiamin (mg)	0.3	0.5	0.7	0.9	1.2	1.4	1.4	1.5	1.4	1.2	1.1	1.1	1.1	1.0	1.0	+0.4	+0.5
Riboflavin (mg)	0.4	0.6	0.8	1.0	1.4	1.6	1.7	1.7	1.6	1.4	1.3	1.3	1.3	1.2	1.2	+0.3	+0.5
Niacin (mg N.E.)¶	6	8	9	11	16	18	18	19	18	16	15	14	14	13	13	+2	+5
Vitamin B_6 (mg)	0.3	0.6	0.9	1.3	1.6	1.8	2.0	2.2	2.2	2.2	1.8	2.0	2.0	2.0	2.0	+0.6	+0.5
Folacin (μg)#	30	45	100	200	300	400	400	400	400	400	400	400	400	400	400	+400	+100
Vitamin B_{12} (μg)**	0.59	1.5	2.0	2.5	3.0	3.0	3.0	3.0	3.0	3.0	3.0	3.0	3.0	3.0	3.0	+1.0	+1.0

Minerals

Calcium (mg)	360	540	800	800	800	1200	1200	800	800	800	1200	1200	800	800	800	+400	+400
Phosphorus (mg)	240	360	800	800	800	1200	1200	800	800	800	1200	1200	800	800	800	+400	+400
Magnesium (mg)	50	70	150	200	250	350	400	350	350	350	300	300	300	300	300	+150	+150
Iron (mg)††	10	15	15	10	10	18	18	10	10	10	18	18	18	18	10	h	h
Zinc (mg)	3	5	10	10	10	15	15	15	15	15	15	15	15	15	15	+5	+10
Iodine (μg)	40	50	70	90	120	150	150	150	150	150	150	150	150	150	150	+25	+50

*The allowances are intended to provide for individual variations among most normal persons as they live in the United States under usual environmental stresses. Diets should be based on a variety of common foods in order to provide other nutrients for which human requirements have been less well defined.

†Retinol equivalents. 1 Retinol equivalent = 1 μg retinol or 6 μg β carotene.

‡As cholecalciferol 10 μg cholecalciferol = 400 I.U. vitamin D.

§α-tocopherol equivalents. 1 mg d-α-tocopherol = 1 α T.E.

¶1 N.E. (niacin equivalent) is equal to 1 mg of niacin or 60 mg of dietary tryptophan.

#The folacin allowances refer to dietary sources as determined by *Lactobacillus casei* assay after treatment with enzymes ("conjugases") to make polyglutamyl forms of the vitamin available to the test organism.

**The RDA for vitamin B₁₂ in infants is based on average concentration of the vitamin in human milk. The allowances after weaning are based on energy intake (as recommended by the American Academy of Pediatrics) and consideration of other factors such as intestinal absorption.

††The increased requirement during pregnancy cannot be met by the iron content of habitual American diets nor by the existing iron stores of many women; therefore the use of 30–60 mg of supplemental iron is recommended. Iron needs during lactation are not substantially different from those of non-pregnant women, but continued supplementation of the mother for 2–3 months after parturition is advisable in order to replenish stores depleted by pregnancy.

(Food and Nutrition Board, National Academy of Sciences–National Research Council, Washington, DC)

Calcium

The daily recommendation for calcium of 1200 mg/day can be met by drinking 960 ml (1 qt) milk every day. Other sources of calcium are other dairy foods (e.g., cheese and yogurt), soft bone, and tofu (soybean curd). Whole or enriched cereal grains and green, leafy vegetables also contain small amounts of calcium.

Sodium

The metabolism of sodium is quite complex and not completely understood. In the past, it was recommended that sodium intake be restricted to avoid the development of preeclampsia, but this restriction has not been proved efficacious. Although routine sodium restriction is not advised, good dietary practices for the general population dictate that salt should be used in moderation. Pregnant patients with chronic hypertension should be placed on a diet with reasonably low sodium intake (2 g).

Other Vitamins and Minerals

Table 7–4 lists the requirements of several vitamins, minerals, and important trace elements. Supplementation with commercially available prenatal vitamins, particularly those that contain extra iron, is advisable, but these supplements must not be substituted for proper food intake. Excessive intake (i.e., 10–90 times the recommended daily allowance) of certain vitamins may be potentially dangerous to the developing fetus (e.g., vitamin A, which may cause bone deformities; vitamin D, which may result in renal pathology; and vitamin C, which may lead to infant dependency).

LACTATION AND THE NURSING MOTHER

Breast milk is the ideal food for all healthy, full-term neonates, as well as for larger, vigorous preterm neonates. A woman's decision to breast-feed depends on many factors, including self-motivation; support by the family, especially the husband; role models; encouragement from physicians and nurses; career plans; and previous experience. With an increasing trend toward breast-feeding, many women who previously would not have considered nursing, such as those with professional careers, are finding time to breast-feed their infants. In addition,

Table 7–4. Recommended Dietary Allowances (Revised 1980)*

Age (yr)	Infants		Children and Adolescents				Adults
	0–0.5	0.5–1	1–3	4–6	7–10	11+	
Vitamins							
Vitamin K (µg)	12	10–20	15–30	20–40	30–60	50–100	70–140
Biotin (µg)	35	50	65	85	120	100–200	100–200
Pantothenic acid (mg)	2	3	3	3–4	4–5	4–7	4–7
Trace Elements†							
Copper (mg)	0.5–0.7	0.7–1.0	1.0–1.5	1.5–2.0	2.0–2.5	2.0–3.0	2.0–3.0
Manganese (mg)	0.5–0.7	0.7–1.0	1.0–1.5	1.5–2.0	2.0–3.0	2.5–5.0	2.5–5.0
Fluoride (mg)	0.1–0.5	0.2–1.0	0.5–1.5	1.0–2.5	1.5–2.5	1.5–2.5	1.5–4.0
Chromium (mg)	0.01–0.04	0.02–0.06	0.02–0.08	0.03–0.12	0.05–0.2	0.05–0.2	0.05–0.2
Selenium (mg)	0.01–0.04	0.02–0.06	0.02–0.08	0.03–0.12	0.05–0.2	0.05–0.2	0.05–0.2
Molybdenum (mg)	0.03–0.06	0.04–0.08	0.05–0.1	0.06–0.15	0.1–0.3	0.15–0.5	0.15–0.5
Electrolytes							
Sodium (mg)	115–350	250–750	325–975	450–1350	600–1800	900–2700	1100–3300
Potassium (mg)	350–925	425–1275	550–1650	775–2325	1000–3000	1525–4575	1875–5625
Chloride (mg)	275–700	400–1200	500–1500	700–2100	925–2775	1400–4200	1700–5100

*Estimates safe and adequate daily dietary intakes of selected vitamins and minerals. Because there is less information on which to base allowances, these figures are not given in the main table of the RDA and are provided here in the form of ranges of recommended intakes.

† Since the toxic levels for many trace elements may be only several times usual intakes, the upper levels for the trace elements given in this table should not be habitually exceeded.

(Food and Nutrition Board, National Academy of Sciences–National Research Council, Washington, DC)

an increasing number of employers are providing day care centers so that women can return to work and continue to nurse their infants.

Mothers who wish to breast-feed should be encouraged enthusiastically to do so. In addition to promoting a more secure maternal-neonatal bond, breast-feeding provides appropriate nutritional benefits for infants; breast milk can be an infant's only source of nutrition for the first 4–6 months of life. At birth, the resistance of the neonate's gastrointestinal tract to various bacterial and viral agents is incompletely developed, and human milk actively prevents these agents from gaining access to the neonate's body. Numerous host resistance factors, such as macrophages, lymphocytes, immunoglobins (especially secretory IgA), lysozyme, lactoferrin, lactoperoxidase, interferon, complement, bifidus factor, and an antistaphylococcal factor are present in large quantities in colostrum. Although the concentration of many of these factors decreases as mature human milk is produced, the infant's ingestion of increased quantities of milk ensures intake of large amounts of these host resistance factors. An intestinal growth-promoting factor similar to that in other mammals has also been identified in human milk. Thus, human milk has been referred to as "nature's vaccine for the newborn." Infants who are breast-fed tend to have a lower incidence of infection and require fewer hospitalizations than infants who are fed formula exclusively.

In families with a strong history of allergy, breast-feeding should be recommended and encouraged, and the ingestion of solid food should be postponed to avoid the introduction of foreign proteins. In rare instances, an infant who is breast-fed may develop symptoms of intestinal intolerance such as colic, abdominal pain, vomiting, or diarrhea. This calls for a careful history of maternal intake and, in most cases, adjustment of the mother's diet rather than discontinuation of nursing.

Since some mothers are discharged less than 12 hours after delivery, there may be little time to acquaint the mother with the techniques of breast-feeding while she is in the hospital. Therefore, it is important that breast-feeding be discussed during the prenatal period; prenatal visits to the pediatrician are of benefit and can be used to reinforce the approach to nursing. Childbirth preparation classes are also an excellent setting for breast-feeding education.

Preparation for Lactation

The mother who plans to breast-feed should begin to prepare her breasts during the last trimester. Any woman, especially one who is fair-haired and light-complexioned, may develop sore, cracked nipples during the first few days or weeks of nursing. If the discomfort is intense or prolonged, the mother may become too discouraged to continue nursing.

The following steps should be taken to toughen the nipples during the third trimester and early postpartum period:

1. Use water only to clean the nipples (i.e., no soap or alcohol).
2. Briskly massage the nipples with a towel when drying after the daily bath or shower. If this results in strong uterine contractions, it may have to be abandoned.
3. Expose the breast frequently to air or allow the bare nipples to rub against outer clothing when at home.

If nipples become cracked during the antepartum or postpartum periods, it may be helpful to apply lanolin or a commercial breast cream twice daily until they are healed. The milk of a mother with cracked nipples may contain a few drops of blood, but this has no known ill effects on the infant.

Nutritional Requirements for Lactation

Lactation places at least as many nutritional demands on a woman as does pregnancy. The nursing mother encounters increased nutritional demands as she requires up to an additional 1000 Kcal/day to feed her offspring during full milk production. If she stores 2–3 kg (4–7 lb) fat during gestation, this provides a reservoir of 14,000–24,000 Kcal for lactation needs. Ordinarily, fat stores will be gradually utilized over the first 4–6 months of nursing.

Without these stores, the nursing mother faces the difficult task of increasing food consumption 50% in order to provide the additional kilocalories required for full milk production.

Protein

The foods selected to provide the increased energy needed for lactation should be of high nutritive value and should contain an additional daily supplement of 20 g protein. High biologic proteins from animal sources should be included in the diet. If the mother is a strict vegetarian, she should be encouraged to make use of a high biologic protein source, and attention should be paid to complementary proteins. Her diet, as well as the growth of her infant, should be carefully monitored.

Vitamins and Minerals

The requirements for various vitamins and minerals increase markedly during lactation. The requirements for vitamin A, vitamin C, and niacin, as well as zinc and iodine, are double those of pregnancy (Table 7–3).

The water-soluble vitamin content of breast milk reflects the mother's intake during lactation. Normally, vitamin C is provided through her fruit and vegetable intake. The B vitamins riboflavin and thiamine are supplied by dairy foods and grains, respectively. The concentration of fat-soluble vitamins in milk is affected only slightly by the mother's diet.

It is important that the mother have good dietary sources of calcium and phosphorus. If dairy foods are not tolerated, soybean milk and supplements such as calcium or soybean curd are required daily. The iron content of mother's milk is not readily affected by her diet. However, iron supplementation replaces iron stores used during pregnancy and lactation.

Trace elements are normally supplied through protein sources and the inclusion of a variety of foods in the diet (Table 7–4). The addition of fluoride to the lactating woman's diet is still a matter of controversy. Concentrations of fluoride found in breast milk are lower than those found in cow's milk, and supplementation of the mother's diet with fluoride has little effect on the fluoride content of her milk.

Hospital Requirements

The hospital should have experienced personnel who can provide emotional support, encouragement, and technical assistance for mothers who wish to nurse their neonates. The personnel should understand the biology of lactation and be flexible about feeding schedules. Often, nursing mothers request rooming-in facilities; this allows the personnel to provide individual instruction in a comfortable setting.

Techniques of Breast-Feeding

Mothers should begin nursing their newborns as soon after delivery as possible. If the mother has received sedation or anesthesia, she may require supervision during this period. The neonate must be kept warm during this process; if skin-to-skin contact is desired, the use of a radiant warmer may be necessary. The staff should arrange for the privacy of the mother and newborn (and often the father) during feeding to make the family comfortable. Feeding schedules should be flexible and should allow for individual biologic variation. The stress of hurried and unpleasant feedings should be avoided. The mother should be allowed to nurse her newborn in any position she and her newborn find comfortable.

Normally, 80–90% of the milk in the breast is ingested during the first 5–7 minutes of nursing. The neonate should begin to suckle on alternate sides, suckling at both breasts during each feeding. To avoid nipple abrasion, cracks, and fissues, it is essential that new mothers be instructed regarding nursing techniques. Particular attention needs to be paid to assuring that during nursing, the nipple and sufficient areola are pulled into the infant's mouth. Remind the mother that breast-feeding entails primarily massaging the areola (and underlying sinus system) which the infant does with lips, gums, and tongue. Suction helps pull the nipple into the correct position but is not the major mechanism of milk flow. The mother should understand that complete and frequent emptying of the breasts produces the maximum amount of milk and also relieves the discomfort of breast engorgement. If the infant appears hungry or is not satisfied with breast-feeding and wants to nurse every 1–2 hours, the mother should permit it. Supplemental formula feedings should be avoided.

Contraindications to Breast-Feeding

There are some contraindications to nursing, but these are encountered infrequently. Mothers with certain chronic illnesses or complications following delivery, such as thrombosis or pulmonary embolism, may not be well enough to nurse their newborns in the immediate neonatal period. The use of anticoagulants, e.g., heparin or dicumarol, is not a contraindication to nursing. A mother with active pulmonary tuberculosis should not nurse. If she is being treated with antituberculous drugs and is culture-negative, however, breast-feeding has been permitted. The mother with an acute cytomegalovirus infection passes the virus to her infant through her milk, and the advisability of breast-feeding in this situation is not clear.

There is great controversy regarding breast-feeding by the mother with hepatitis B virus. The follow-up of infants of mothers with hepatitis B reveals that the surface antigen is present in approximately 35–50% of their infants by 4–6 months of age whether or not the mother breast-feeds. Several authorities insist that these mothers should be discouraged from breast-feeding, but the data to support these recommendations are uncertain.

A mother who has active infection with herpes simplex virus may breast-feed her infant if she follows very careful hand-washing procedures and takes meticulous care to ensure that the infant is not exposed directly to the lesions. This may be very difficult for some mothers to accomplish, and breast-feeding may have to be discouraged in these particular situations.

Maternal Medications and Nursing

The effect of drugs taken by the mother on the nursing infant is controversial. Unfortunately, much that has been written regarding the excretion of drugs in milk is based on insufficient data. However, several excellent recent reviews indicate that few drugs taken by the mother require her to discontinue breast-feeding. It is important for the mother to discuss the use of medications with her obstetrician and pediatrician if she wishes to continue breast-feeding. In such situations, the infant should be carefully followed to detect any adverse effects.

One of the most pressing unanswered questions is the effect of pollutants, including pesticides, that are excreted in breast milk. The concentration of pesticides in breast milk varies from region to region, and no general recommendations regarding breast-feeding by women with specific concentrations of pesticides in their milk currently can be made with a firm scientific basis. State health departments may be consulted.

Other problems encountered with breast-feeding involve infants who develop breast milk jaundice (see Chapter 10) or who have an inborn error of amino acid metabolism. Certainly, infants with galactosemia should not be breast-fed; they must be given formula that contains neither lactose nor galactose. Similarly, infants whith phenylketonuria require a formula such as Lofenalac, although they may also be able to tolerate small amounts of breast milk.

Breast Milk for Sick or Preterm Neonates

Many mothers wish to provide breast milk for their sick or preterm neonates and should be encouraged to do so. They should be instructed in techniques of milk collection in order to prevent contamination and overgrowth of bacteria. Careful hand-washing techniques and wiping of the breast with cotton pledgets prior to collection are of paramount importance. The first 5–10 ml of milk contain the greatest number of bacteria and should be discarded. In a sense, a "midstream" milk should be collected. It has been recommended that plastic containers be used instead of glass containers, because the cells of human milk tend to cling to glass and are thus not available for the neonate. If the milk is refrigerated for longer than 12 hours, however, the numbers of cells in glass or plastic containers are almost identical. If the milk can be used within 24–48 hours, refrigeration is adequate. If a longer period is to pass before the milk is given to the neonate, the milk should be frozen. Mothers who live great distances from the hospital in which their neonate is cared for may have to freeze their milk before it is transported to the medical center. In such cases, freshly expressed milk should be refrigerated before it is added to the frozen pool to prevent frequent rethawing of frozen milk.

Freshly expressed human milk has an advantage over processed milk in that many of the cells and certainly the host resistance factors are available to the neonate in an unaltered state. Freezing and thawing destroy the cells and probably slightly decrease the concentrations of the immunoglobins. Even when milk is processed by the Holder technique (62°–65° C for 30 minutes), the host resistance factors are decreased by at least 25–30%. Terminal sterilization of human milk is not recommended because it destroys all the cells and most of the host resistance factors.

FORMULA FEEDING

If a mother desires to feed formula to her newborn her decision should be supported by physicians and nursing staff. She certainly should not be made to feel inadequate because she does not choose to breast-feed. Flexible feeding schedules should be utilized. Formula-fed neonates should be fed by their mothers; propping of the bottle by any method whatsoever is to be condemned. Like breast-feeding mothers, those women who wish to bottle-feed their newborn should wash their hands carefully and should feed their newborn in a comfortable position.

Formula selection and control should be a physician-directed activity. New formulas should be reviewed by the appropriate hospital committees and the director of the nursery before use.

The hospital should have written policies regarding the use of formulas in the nursery; appropriate information regarding composition, preparation, distribution, and control should be included. The physician should write orders for the formula to be used and the amount to be given at each feeding.

The composition of formulas currently used in many nurseries is listed in Table 7–5. Data on the type and amounts of protein, fat, and carbohydrate, as well as the concentration of sodium, potassium, phosphorus, and calcium, have been provided by the manufacturer, but values may vary slightly from one lot to the next.

Table 7–5. *Source and Composition of Infant Formulas*

Formula/milk	Calories/oz	Protein Source	g/dl	Fat Source	g/dl	Carbohydrate Source	g/dl	Na (mEq/liter)	K (mEq/liter)	Phosphorus (mg/dl)	Calcium (mg/dl)	Osmolality (Osm/kg water)
						Feeding at Infancy						
Human milk	20	Human milk	1.0–1.2	Human milk	4.5	Lactose	7.0	7	13	16	34	300
Enfamil	20	Skim milk	1.5	Soy oil, coconut oil	3.7	Lactose	7.0	12	18	46	55	290
Enfamil Premature	24	Whey, casein	2.4	MCT, corn oil	4.1	Lactose, corn syrup solids	8.9	14	23	48	95	396
Isomil	20	Soy protein isolate with L-methionine	2.0	Soy oil, coconut oil	3.6	Corn syrup, sucrose	6.8	13	18	50	70	256
Lofenalac	20	Casein hydrolysate	2.2	Corn oil	2.7	Corn syrup solids, tapioca starch	8.7	14	17	47	63	454
Lonalac	20	Casein	3.4	Coconut oil	3.5	Lactose	4.8	1.1	26	100	110	241
Meat base	20	Beef hearts	2.8	Sesame oil	3.3	Cane sugar, tapioca	6.2	8	10	65	99	289
Nursoy	20	Soy isolate with L-methionine	2.1	Oleo, coconut oil, olein, Soy	3.6	Sucrose	6.9	8	18	42	60	296
Nutramigen	20	Casein hydrolysate	2.2	Corn oil	2.6	Sucrose, tapioca starch	8.8	14	17	47	63	443
Portagen	20	Casein	2.4	MCT, corn oil	3.2	Corn syrup solids, sucrose, lactose	7.8	14	22	47	63	236

Product											
Pregestimil	20	Casein hydrolysate	1.9	MCT, corn oil	2.7	Tapioca starch, corn syrup solids	9.1	14	18	42	63	335
Prosobee	20	Soy protein isolate with L-methionine	2.0	Soy oil, coconut oil	3.6	Corn syrup solids	6.9	12	17	47	60	160
Similac	20	Skim milk	1.6	Coconut oil, soy oil	3.6	Lactose	7.2	11	20	39	51	290
Similac PM 60/40	20	Whey, casein	1.6	Coconut oil, corn oil	3.7	Lactose	6.9	7	15	20	40	266
Similac—LBW	24	Skim milk	2.2	MCT, coconut oil, soy oil	4.5	Lactose, corn syrup solids	8.5	16	26	56	78	300
Similac Special Care	24	Whey, casein	2.2	MCT, corn oil, coconut oil	4.4	Lactose, corn syrup solids	8.6	15	26	72	144	300
SMA	20	Whey, casein	1.5	Oleo, coconut oil, safflower oil, soy oil	3.5	Lactose	7.2	6	14	33	44	300
SMA Preemie	24	Whey, casein	2.0	Oleo, coconut oil, olein, soy MCT	4.4	Lactose, maltodextrins	8.6	14	19	40	75	268
Soyalac	20	Soybean, solids	2.1	Soy oil	3.7	Sucrose, corn syrup solids	6.6	13	19	50	60	210
I-Soyalac	20	Soy protein isolate with L-methionine	2.1	Soy oil	3.7	Sucrose, tapioca starch	6.6	16	18	50	60	230
Advanced Feeding Beyond Infancy											
Similac Advance	16	Cow's milk, soy protein	2.0	Soy oil, corn oil	2.7	Corn syrup, lactose	5.5	13	22	23	26	210
Cow's milk	20	Cow's milk	3.3	Cow's milk	3.7	Lactose	4.8	25	35	95	124	233

At present, few hospitals prepare their own formula for the routine feeding of normal neonates although some hospitals use dietary kitchens or the hospital pharmacy to prepare special formulas. Recommendations for formula room construction and facilities are available from the American Hospital Association.

Presterilized Ready-to-Feed Formulas in Individual Nursing Units

Most hospitals now utilize prepared nursing units with separate nipples that are readily attached to the bottles just before use. These nursing units may be stored in any convenient, clean, cool area; refrigeration is not necessary. Sufficient formula for a 24-hour period should be on hand. The area in which nipples are uncapped and placed on the bottle must be kept scrupulously clean and must be used only for formula preparation. The sterile cap should be kept on the nipple until the formula is ready to be given to the neonate. Nipples may be uncapped and attached to bottles at the mother's bedside just prior to feeding. Disposable nipples should not be reused. The formula should be used within 4 hours after the bottle is uncapped.

Presterilized Formulas in Bulk Containers

Formulas in a powder form are provided in bulk containers that do not require refrigeration. The formula may be made up in the area that is used for capping and uncapping. Usually, the powder is added to sterile water in prescribed quantities, gently shaken to make sure that the powder is completely dissolved, and fed to the neonate. Similarly, formulas can be mixed by diluting concentrated liquid preparations. Containers of liquid formulas should be discarded if they have been opened for longer than 4 hours.

Standards of control must be followed if formulas are being prepared in the nursery. As stated, a special area must be designated for this use, and continuous bacteriologic testing of samples from the nursing unit should be done.

VITAMIN AND MINERAL SUPPLEMENTATION

Infants who are breast-fed may show evidence of vitamin D deficiency if their mothers have low vitamin D intakes or little exposure to sunlight, either antepartum or postpartum. If there is a possibility that the mother's vitamin D status is not optimal, the infant fed human milk should receive 400 IU/day supplemental vitamin D. This may be of particular importance for dark-skinned infants and for those situations in which exposure to sunshine is very limited. When sun exposure can safely be recommended, supplemental vitamin D may not be necessary.

Fluoride supplementation is still a matter of controversy. The AAP Committee on Nutrition recommends initiating fluoride supplements in breast-fed infants shortly after birth, but also recognizes that fluoride supplementation could be initiated at 6 months of age.

The iron content of human milk is low, but the bioavailability is such that approximately 50% of the iron is absorbed. It is recommended that the infants who are exclusively breast-fed be given supplemental iron when they reach 4–6 months of age. Vitamins and minerals have been added to commercial formula, and supplementation is not necessary when formulas containing 12 mg/dl iron are used. It has been alleged that some infants fed iron-containing formulas have exhibited colic and other gastrointestinal symptoms. In carefully controlled studies, however, these observations were not verified.

Preterm neonates do not require iron supplementation until they begin to grow rapidly, usually 2–6 weeks after delivery. At that time, iron supplementation should be given, but it is important that vitamin E be adequate. Iron supplementation in an infant who is deficient in vitamin E may lead to hemolytic anemia.

The diet of preterm neonates should be supplemented with vitamins. Those who are receiving human milk or formula should also be given vitamin supplementation, because the concentration of vitamins in the small amount of milk that they ingest is not adequate. Each day, the neonate should receive 20–50 mg vitamin C, 400 units vitamin D, and 5–10 IU vitamin E. Preterm neonates do not absorb folate well, and 50–100 μg/day supplemental folic acid are recommended for these neonates, beginning at approximately 2 weeks of age.

FEEDING LOW-BIRTH-WEIGHT AND SICK NEONATES

Because of the immaturity of their gastrointestinal tract, prematurely born neonates often cannot tolerate oral feeding. Intravenous glucose and water should be initiated within the first hours after birth. The intricacies of intravenous feedings have been discussed in several publications.

At the end of the first week of postnatal life, an attempt should be made to provide at least 60 Kcal/kg/day. There is a tendency to give excessive amounts of amino acids at this time. There is also a tendency to give sick, low-birth-weight neonates excessive amounts of fluids. These neonates have a higher than normal level of body water at birth and often have excessive lung fluid as well. Fluid therapy should not be governed by "rules of thumb," but should be determined by calculations of the neonate's clinical and biochemical status at 8- to 12-hour intervals. The initial fluid intake in distressed neonates cared for in conventional incubators should be close to basal requirements (40–50 ml/kg/day) and subsequently increased as indicated. Neonates who are being cared for under radiant warmers or who are receiving phototherapy often require more fluid to supplement increased insensible water loss.

The parenteral nutrition fluids should be prepared in the pharmacy under laminar flow hood conditions with sterile technique. Such mixtures should not be prepared in the nursery. Careful monitoring of the neonate's blood gases, electrolytes, and chemistries is important in order to avoid complications that may occur with the use of parenteral nutrition. After the intravenous feedings are initiated, oral feedings can be gradually introduced as the neonate is adapting to extrauterine life.

The amount per feeding that can be given without overloading the immature gastrointestinal tract depends on the weight, maturity, and condition of the neonate. Neonates with cardiopulmonary disease tolerate feeding poorly, for example. Their initial feeding is usually 2 ml/kg, and the volume is increased slowly over time, as tolerated. Most centers use either orogastric or nasogastric bolus feedings. Continuous feeding by means of nasogastric or orogastric tubes has also been used, and there is increasing evidence that such feedings are better tolerated and that absorption is improved in many neonates. Because gastric emptying time is delayed and the gastroesophageal sphincter is often incompetent, reflux is frequently encountered in the low-birth-weight neonate. Transpyloric feeding with the use of Silastic, polyurethane, or Silicone rubber tubes may be necessary for such neonates. If continuous feedings are used, not more than 24 hours' supply should be provided in the tubing. Allowing the milk to remain for longer periods may increase the incidence of contamination and may lead to infection in the neonate. Personnel should give meticulous attention to hand-washing before mixing and hanging formulas, and careful bacteriologic monitoring should be initiated.

No matter what types of feedings are used, these neonates should be monitored carefully in order to detect early signs of abdominal distention. Gastric residuals should be monitored, and stools should be tested intermittently to detect microscopic bleeding. Hypertonic feedings should be avoided, especially during the first several weeks of life, in order to avoid complications such as necrotizing enterocolitis or lactobezoars.

The neonate who is small for gestational age is at great risk of developing complications such as hypoglycemia, hypocalcemia, and polycythemia. Such a neonate often tolerates oral feedings poorly. These problems should be anticipated and avoided. In many instances, the neonate should be started on intravenous feedings until it can be shown that the neonate can maintain a normal blood glucose level and tolerate oral feedings.

NUTRITIONAL COUNSELING

Ideally, a nutritional counseling program should be available in each center that provides perinatal care. Persons knowledgeable in perinatal nutrition can greatly enhance the parents' knowledge regarding their own nutrition as well as that of their newborn. Specialized programs for unusual and difficult nutritional disorders should be available for those who desire or need them.

RESOURCES AND RECOMMENDED READING

American Academy of Pediatrics, Committee on Drugs: The Excretion of Drugs in Breat Milk. In press

American Academy of Pediatrics, Committee on Nutrition: Fluoride supplementation: Revised dosage schedule. Pediatrics 63:150–152, 1979

American College of Obstetricians and Gynecologists: Assessment of Maternal Nutrition. Washington, DC, ACOG, 1978 (revised edition, 1982)

American College of Obstetricians and Gynecologists: Nutrition in Maternal Health Care. Washington, DC, ACOG, 1974

American Hospital Association: Procedures and Layout for the Infant Formula Room, Chicago, AHA, 1965

Be Good to Your Baby Before It Is Born. White Plains, NY, March of Dimes–Birth Defects Foundation, 1977

Catz CS, Giacoia GP: Drugs and breast milk. Pediatr Clin North Am 19(1):151–166, 1972

Committee on Nutrition of the Mother and Preschool Child: Nutritional Services in Perinatal Care. Washington, DC, National Academy Press, 1981

Ernest AE, McCabe ERB, Neifert MR, et al: Guide to breast feeding the infant with PKU. US Department of Health and Human Services, Publication No. (HSA) 79-5110. Washington, DC, US Government Printing Office, 1980

Jelliffe DB, Jelliffe EFP: Human Milk in the Modern World: Psychosocial, nutritional and economic significance. Oxford, Oxford University Press, 1981

Lawrence RA: Breast-feeding: A guide for the medical profession. St Louis, CV Mosby, 1980

Luke B: Maternal Nutrition. Boston, Little, Brown, 1979, pp 183–195

Stagno S, Reynolds DW, Pass RF, et al: Breast milk and the risk of cytomegalovirus infection. N Engl J Med 302(19):1073–1076, 1980

U.S. Department of Health, Education, and Welfare; Public Health Service; Health Services Administration: Food for the Teenager During Pregnancy. DHEW Publication No. (HSA) 76-5611. Washington, DC, US Government Printing Office, 1976 chapter **8**

Interhospital Care of the Perinatal Patient

The transport of pregnant women, mothers, and neonates between hospitals is a recognized and essential component of modern perinatal care. As noted in Chapter 1, transportation is one of the systems approaches to obstetric and newborn care. There are three types of patient transport: maternal-fetal, neonatal, and return.

Maternal-fetal transports involve pregnant women who are to be admitted for delivery, unlike obstetric consultations, which involve ambulatory evaluation without admission. Neonatal transports usually employ a team to evaluate and stabilize the neonate's condition, as well as to provide care when indicated. Return transports take patients back to their original or local hospital for further care when the problems that required transport have been resolved. Return transports should be recognized as an important benefit to the individual patient and system.

The Committee on the Fetus and Newborn of the American Academy of Pediatrics has established a policy on Level II neonatal units, stating that "Level II neonatal units must have ongoing liaison with a Level III neonatal intensive care unit." That firm support for a network can logically be extended to all perinatal services. The referral of high-risk mothers, as well as sick newborns, to regional centers for care has a positive impact on local perinatal care and makes it necessary to set guidelines for regional perinatal networks. The rising costs of care, the ascending expectations of consumers, and the constraints on spending are relevant considerations in a movement toward firmer guidelines for interhospital care of the perinatal patient.

Interhospital transport and care of high-risk perinatal patients make it reasonable to expect that every patient in a region will be cared for in an appropriate manner. A successful program of interhospital care should incorporate the following components:

1. Risk identification, which includes active anticipation of needs that will require the movement of patients in order to provide optimum care

2. Recognition that patient care is a continuous process

3. Local physicians who know the resources that are available and how to gain access to them

4. Physicians at all levels who have the knowledge and skills needed to identify the high-risk patient, to evaluate the patient's condition, and to stabilize and prepare the patient for transfer

5. An organized, appropriate, and available interhospital transport service

6. A political and economic environment that provides support for the interhospital transport system

7. Data collection and analysis for purposes of monitoring and evaluating the program

From the moment a perinatal problem is recognized, to the point of its resolution and follow-up, there should be a continuum of care. Because disease processes do not become static while a patient is being transferred, management is necessary during transport. The objective of interhospital care thus becomes the provision of the maximum degree of care possible within the constraints imposed by a moving ambulance, its restricted space, and its lack of support facilities (e.g., laboratory, blood bank, and radiology services).

INDICATIONS FOR TRANSPORT

The circumstances in which patients are transported vary according to the distribution of care facilities in each region. The decision should be made by the initial physician and a consultant, both of whom should be well-informed of the resources at each center. In general, transport should be considered when the resources immediately available to the maternal, fetal, or neonatal patient are not adequate to deal with the patient's actual or predicted medical or surgical complications.

The following patient conditions require more specialized care and may require patient transfer. The specific values are to be considered guidelines only. They will vary with individual patient needs or institutional capabilities.

I. Maternal Conditions
    A. Obstetric complications
        1. Premature rupture of membranes (at less than 34 weeks' gestation or less than 2000 g expected birth weight)
        2. Premature labor (at less than 34 weeks' gestation or less than 2000 g expected birth weight)
        3. Any condition creating the probability of birth at less than 34 weeks' gestation or less than 2000 g expected birth weight
            a. Severe preeclampsia or other hypertensive complication
            b. Multiple gestation
            c. Intrauterine growth retardation
            d. Third trimester bleeding
            e. Rh isoimmunization
            f. Premature dilation of the cervix
    B. Medical complications
        1. Infections in which the degree or nature of maternal illness may result in premature birth
            a. Hepatitis
            b. Pyelonephritis
            c. Influenza
            d. Pneumonia
            e. Other febrile or hypermetabolic conditions
        2. Severe organic heart disease, functional class III or IV
        3. Poorly controlled diabetes mellitus
        4. Thyrotoxicosis
        5. Renal disease with deteriorating function or increased hypertension
        6. Drug overdose
        7. Miscellaneous severe illnesses
    C. Surgical complications
        1. Trauma requiring intensive care or surgical correction beyond the capabilities of local facilities or where the procedure may result in the onset of premature labor
        2. Acute abdominal emergencies at less than 34 weeks' gestation or with a fetus weighing less than 2000 g
        3. Thoracic emergencies requiring intensive care or surgical correction
II. Neonatal Conditions
    A. Gestation less than 34 weeks or weight less than 2000 g
    B. Neonatal sepsis or infection

C. Respiratory distress and metabolic acidosis persisting after 2 hours of age
D. Neonatal blood loss
E. Hypoglycemia
F. Hemolytic disease of the newborn
G. Neonates of mothers taking hazardous drugs
H. Neonates of diabetic mothers
I. Neonatal seizures
J. Sepsis or meningitis
K. Congenital malformations requiring surgical care or observation
L. Shock or asphyxia persisting beyond 2 hours
M. Neonatal cardiac disorders with persisting cyanosis
N. Progressive, increasing respiratory distress syndrome
O. Any neonatal condition requiring ventilatory support for more than 1 hour
P. Neonates needing more than routine observation or care

THE ORGANIZED APPROACH TO TRANSPORT

The provision of adequate life support during the transport of critically ill mothers and neonates requires considerable knowledge, skill, experience, and specialized equipment not readily available in all hospitals. Many perinatal centers that provide Level III services have developed transport systems for their service regions because only experience with a large number of patients can maintain the skills required for care during transport. The referring staff can help the mother and neonate most by calling for assistance as soon as the need for transport becomes apparent and by using the time before transport to stabilize the patients and prepare for transport. This practice ameliorates the immediate problems and reduces the time that the transport team must be in the referring hospital.

In certain circumstances, it is reasonable for the referring physician to manage the transfer personally. Maternal-fetal transports are frequently conducted in this fashion. The procedure whereby transport originates at the referring hospital, frequently termed one-way transport, functions effectively in some locations; however, two-way transport systems, which operate from a base at the center, are more common. Any transport procedure is acceptable if the guidelines given here are utilized and its goals and objectives are attained.

Informal, poorly organized interhospital care is hazardous. In order to avoid compromising the patient, to ensure a predictable response for transportation requests, and to provide the highest quality of care, the approach to transport must be logical and organized. When the number of patients who require interhospital care is small, efforts to monitor and maintain the skill levels of the team become even more important. It is advisable in such instances to consider the consolidation of care programs.

An interhospital care system has five identifiable components: (1) organization, (2) communications, (3) personnel, (4) equipment, and (5) transport vehicles.

Organization

Interhospital care should be available 24 hours/day, in a program with defined response time and minimum capabilities of personnel. The director should be a specialist in maternal-fetal medicine or neonatal medicine, or a board-certified pediatrician or obstetrician with a special interest in these subspecialty areas. The director's responsibilities are:

1. Quality control of patient care through regular case review
2. Personnel training and supervision
3. Development and utilization of patient care protocols
4. Development and utilization of record-keeping systems and subsequent collation and evaluation of data for analysis
5. Review of operational aspects, e.g., response times, effectiveness of communications, and equipment maintenance

Communications

The transfer of a patient from one hospital to another and from one care team to another requires a reliable communications system. It is essential that the referring physician provide the receiving physician with specific clinical information on the patient being referred. For a maternal patient, the following information should be included:

Reason for admission
Age
Date of last menstrual period
Estimated date of confinement
Gravida, para, and abortion
Relevant health problems
Perinatal history

Blood type
Results of amniocentesis
Reasons for transfer
Therapy administered, including drugs
Intake and output

For a neonatal patient, the following information should be included:

Gestational age and weight
Perinatal history
Temperature
Color
Hematocrit
Oxygen requirement and blood gas levels
Respiratory activity (particularly presence of apnea or need for assisted ventilation)
Blood glucose or Dextrostix
Pertinent radiologic findings
Reasons for transfer
Therapy administered, including drugs

This information allows the receiving facility to prepare for the patient's stabilization, transfer, and admission. Appendixes F and G contain sample record formats for information that can be provided conveniently by telephone. For large service areas, toll-free lines should be established by the referral center for referring physicians and families. In metropolitan areas or over short distances, direct hotlines may link referring obstetric units and nurseries to the center. These lines should be open 24 hours/day and should be well publicized throughout the service region. The liaison between the referring and the receiving centers should include telephone or radio communication during stabilization and transfer.

Appropriate historical data should accompany the patient. This information should include appropriate laboratory data and x-rays. In most neonatal transports, 10 ml clotted maternal blood to be used for cross-matching purposes should be obtained and should accompany the transport team. Cord blood and the placenta may be helpful in certain clinical situations, such as multiple gestation or intrauterine growth retardation.

Dispatching services should provide rapid coordination of vehicles and personnel, as well as communication links between referring and receiving hospitals and the transfer team. Referring physicians should be given an estimated arrival time to allow them to arrange for laboratory studies on which to base therapy in transport and ensure their availability at the time of transport. The receiving hospital should also be given an estimated arrival time to allow the staff to prepare for the patient's arrival. When flights must connect with ground ambulances, it is desirable for a single dispatching center to coordinate the movements of all vehicles. The complexity and sophistication of the dispatching operation vary considerably with the nature of the service.

Personnel

The interhospital care team members should have the collective expertise sufficient to provide the necessary supportive care for a wide variety of emergency conditions in high-risk mothers and neonates. Team members may be drawn from appropriately trained physicians, registered nurses, respiratory therapists, and emergency medical technicians. One member should usually be a physician or registered nurse. Neonatal nurse-clinicians are often specifically identified with this role. In addition to being highly knowledgeable in care and procedures for perinatal patients, transport personnel should be thoroughly familiar with transport equipment; any malfunction en route must be managed without the assistance of hospital maintenance staff.

Equipment

Powered equipment should have "stand alone" capability, i.e., it should be battery-operated. Batteries should have sufficient power to operate the equipment for the duration of the transport if no alternative power source is available. Furthermore, critical equipment should be adaptable to 12- and 24-volt DC and 110-volt AC power for use in a hospital or ambulance.

In addition to equipment for monitoring, resuscitation, and support of both mother and neonate, a transport kit containing essential drugs and special supplies should be continuously available during stabilization and transfer of the patient. A list of equipment and drugs that should be included in a transport kit is found in Appendix H.

Transport Vehicles

The main concern during transport is to maintain optimum care. The choice of a ground or air ambulance is based on distance from one hospital to another and facilities available to support the patient during the transfer. Ground ambulances are most useful for distances up to 80–100 miles of flat terrain in low traffic density areas. Beyond 100 miles, aircraft may be faster or less expensive, even though ground ambulances provide more direct transfer between regional centers. The pressurization of aircraft is an important consideration during management, since adequate oxygen levels of the mother and fetus or newborn must be ensured.

Helicopters are used in some areas to transport patients up to a few hundred miles or to reach patients in difficult terrain or high traffic density areas. Helicopters are not pressurized, are generally noisier and more confined, and have less range than fixed wing aircraft, however. These limitations should be considered whenever a helicopter is used.

TRANSPORT PROCEDURE

Evaluation

The patient's condition should be carefully evaluated at the referring hospital, both in regard to the primary diagnosis and the presence of complicating conditions. Steps should be taken to correct these conditions to the extent possible prior to transfer.

Stabilization

Transport of the maternal patient may require hemodynamic stabilization; the initiation of tocolytic agents, anticonvulsants, or antihypertension agents; or demonstrated arrest or diminution of active labor. Patients with active bleeding, rapidly progressive preeclampsia, and rapidly progressive labor should not be transported until appropriate medical management has been initiated and, in the opinion of the medical team, the possibility of acute crisis or delivery in transport is significantly diminished. In some situations, maternal transport may not be advisable; it may be preferable to coordinate neonate transport in such a fashion that the transport team arrives at the referring hospital immediately prior to or shortly after the birth. Transport teams may, by prior agreement between the referring physician and the dispatch center, participate in the initial stabilization at birth. In the fully stabilized neonate, temperature, blood gas levels, blood pressure, tissue perfusion, and blood glucose level are normal. Complete stabilization of a newborn is not always possible, but transport of an extremely unstable newborn is contraindicated.

Although there have been no controlled trials, experience indicates that stabilization prior to departure is probably the most critical aspect of interhospital care because it minimizes subsequent deterioration in an environment that may not permit detection or treatment of problems.

Medicolegal Concerns

There are many legal considerations in perinatal transport. Many details are not well defined, but all involved parties, including the referring hospital and personnel, the receiving hospital and personnel, and commercial ambulance and aircraft charter corporations, assume responsibilities. As spokesperson for the transport team, the physician should thoroughly explain to the patient or the parents of the newborn the patient's condition and reasons for transfer. Informed consent for transfer, admission, and care should be obtained. The newborn should be clearly identified.

Perinatal transport teams are involved in very special transport situations, and prior attention to potential legal problems is advised. In most situations, the institution that employs the team is responsible for its actions, and professional duties are performed under the direction and authority of a physician-director at the receiving hospital. Many hospitals consider neonates admitted to their institution while en route and under the care of the transport team. Physician-directors and hospital administrators should recognize the potential administrative or legal problems that may arise in certain situations, for example, when transport teams cross one or more state lines during a transport.

The referring physician preferably should remain at the hospital until the neonatal transport team arrives and should be there while the team is present in order to ensure complete communication. The patient must pass from the official care of the referring physician to that of the transport team at some point; the departure of the transport team from the physical premises of the referring hospital might be considered the official point of transfer of responsibility. Individual hospitals and regions should investigate the use of transfer agreements, which might include granting of emergency privileges to members of transport teams.

The referral center should receive a report on the patient's condition prior to departure. In the case of newborn transport, the mother and father should be offered the opportunity to see and touch the neonate before the transfer, even if the neonate is in a transport incubator or on a respirator. In addition, an instant picture of the neonate may be taken for the family prior to transport. This has proved particularly helpful when parents and their neonates are to be separated for a long period or when the mother is recovering from a cesarean delivery and may not remember the time spent with the neonate prior to transport. The family of the patient should also receive written information about the receiving hospital, names of staff members, visiting hours, telephone numbers, and places to stay in the vicinity of the hospital. Brochures about the hospital can be helpful. A desire to breast-feed should be reinforced, and the mother should be taught how to express milk until nipple feeding becomes possible. Early attention to family needs and concerns at this critical time can reduce anxiety and ease the transition to a new medical center.

Records are essential for the continuing care of the patient and for the evaluation of the referral transport process. Records should include the following information:

Patient's name

Referring hospital

Receiving hospital

Referring physician

Attendants' names and professional status

Mode of transport

Time data, including arrival at the referring hospital, departure, ground or air ambulance time, and arrival at the receiving hospital

Patient's age, weight, gestational age, and sex

Diagnosis and condition

Procedures performed

Medication administered

Periodic vital signs

Special comments

PATIENT CARE IN TRANSIT

A well-stabilized patient requires little or no intervention during transport. The patient should be under continuous observation, however. The key factors to be monitored in the maternal patient include blood pressure, uterine contractions, cervical dilation, fetal heart rate ultrasonography, deep tendon reflexes, infusion rate of intravenous fluids, and the administration of tocolytic agents or anticonvulsants. For the newborn, temperature, respiration, heart rate, blood pressure, color, activity, and oxygen concentration should be monitored frequently by noninvasive means. A neutral thermal environment should be maintained. It may be necessary to monitor other parameters as well, such as the blood glucose level. Monitoring of blood gases during transport is feasible with the availability of portable transcutaneous monitoring.

The patient, attending personnel, and all equipment should be safely secured in the transport vehicle. Although it may be necessary to respond rapidly to an emergency, high-speed ground travel greatly increases the risk of accidents. In the majority of cases, there is little need for excessive speed if the patient is stabilized.

RECEIVING AND COMPLETING TRANSFER

The receiving staff should be prepared to deal with any unresolved problems or emergencies. The patient's history and clinical status, as well as all the plans for current management, should be communicated directly by the transport personnel. Therapies provided during transport should not be changed unless the transport team is consulted.

Family members are extremely anxious when a patient is transferred. If they have not been able to accompany or follow the patient, they should be called as soon as possible after the transfer and given a report on the patient's condition. The referring physician and the nursing staff at the referring hospital should also be informed about the patient's arrival at the receiving hospital and the patient's progress on a continuing basis thereafter.

The transfer is not complete until equipment on the transport vehicle has been restocked and prepared for the next call. Reusable equipment that has come into contact with the patient should be appropriately sterilized or decontaminated.

OUTREACH EDUCATION AND THE REGIONAL TRANSPORT SYSTEM

Since interhospital care of the high-risk perinatal patient requires the cooperation and coordination of many skilled persons, outreach education efforts should include discussions of the regional transport system. Outreach education can be used to reinforce that cooperation and coordination.

Outreach education related to transport should focus on the following objectives:

1. Informing perinatal care providers in the region of the specialized resources available to them through the perinatal network
2. Assisting primary physicians in developing their abilities to anticipate complications, to identify high-risk perinatal patients, and to stabilize these patients before transport
3. Facilitating effective quality assurance through the continuing education of perinatal care providers
4. Establishing 24-hour consultation and referral sources
5. Promoting a regionalized care system designed to ensure high-quality care to all patients in a cost-efficient fashion

PLANNING AND EVALUATION

The planning of the perinatal transport system requires the participation of both those who will use the service and those who will provide it. The creation of regional advisory councils with representatives from the various perinatal programs facilitates planning and evaluation, as such a group can identify and verify the particular region's needs for interhospital perinatal transport and the specific characteristics of the service that should be designed in response to those needs. The characteristics of the successful system, as described earlier, can be used as a guide for program development and subsequent evaluation. Other criteria should be considered in planning and evaluating the transport system:

1. Availability: Does the system provide all services that may be needed by the perinatal patient?
2. Accessibility: Is the capacity to "connect" the patient quickly and appropriately with the services needed ensured? Do those who will need the services know where to go to get them?
3. Responsiveness: Is there a mutual commitment from referring care providers and specialized care providers to honor and accommodate each other's special needs as they may arise?
4. Effectiveness: Are perinatal patients being given the appropriate care in the appropriate setting? Do care users, physicians and patients, and care providers regard the perinatal transport service as useful and effective?

As basic as these questions may appear, their answers are often assumed without testing. The purpose of the evaluation of the system is to collect the evidence that will confirm that the system provides high-quality care to high-risk mothers and neonates.

RESOURCES AND RECOMMENDED READING

Boehm FH, Haire MF: One-way maternal transport: An evolving concept in patient services. Am J Obstet Gynecol 134(4):484–492, 1979

Butterfield LJ: Evaluation and economic exigency in the NICU, editorial. N Engl J Med 305(9):518–519, 1981

Chance GW, O'Brien MJ, Swyer PR: Transportation of sick neonates, 1972: An unsatisfactory aspect of medical care. Can Med Assoc J 109(9):847–851, 1973

Ferrara A, Harin A: Emergency Transfer of the High-Risk Neonate: A working manual for medical, nursing and administrative personnel. St. Louis, CV Mosby, 1980.

Giles HR, Isaman J, Moore WJ, et al: The Arizona high-risk maternal transport system: An initial view. Am J Obstet Gynecol 128(4):400–407, 1977

Harris TB, Isamen J, Giles HR: Improved neonatal survival through maternal transport. Obstet Gynecol 52(3):294–300, 1978

Mead Johnson & Co., Nutritional Division: Maternal Air Transport. Conference proceedings, Denver, March 1979. Evanston, IN, Mead Johnson & Co., 1979

Mead Johnson & Co., Nutritional Division: Newborn Air Transport. Conference Proceedings, Denver, February 1978. Evansville, IN, Mead Johnson & Co., 1978

Merenstein GB, Pettett G, Woodall J, et al: An analysis of air transport results in the sick newborn: II. Antenatal and neonatal referrals. Am J. Obstet Gynecol 128(5):520–525, 1977

Modanlou HD, Dorchester W, Freeman RK, et al: Perinatal transport to a regional perinatal center in a metropolitan area: Maternal versus neonatal transport. Am J Obstet Gynecol 138(8):1157–1164, 1980

Modanlou HD, Dorchester WS, Thorosian A, et al: Antenatal versus neonatal transport to a regional perinatal center: A comparison between matched pairs. Obstet Gynecol 53(6):725–729, 1979

National Foundation–March of Dimes, Committee on Perinatal Health: Toward Improving the Outcome of Pregnancy. White Plains, NY, National Foundation–March of Dimes, 1976

Pettet G, et al: An analysis of air transport results in the sick newborn infant: I. The transport team. Pediatrics 55(6):774–782, 1975

Phillip AGS, Little GA, Polivy DR, et al: Neonatal mortality risk for the eighties: The importance of birthweight/gestational age groups. Pediatrics 68(1):122–130, 1981

Segal S (ed): Manual for the Transport of High-Risk Newborn Infants: Principles, policies, equipment, techniques. Vancouver, Canadian Pediatric Society, 1972

Sinclair JC, Torrance GW, Boyle MH, et al: Evaluation of neonatal-intensive-care programs. N Engl J Med 305(9):489–494, 1981 chapter

9

Evaluation of Perinatal Care

Evaluation of perinatal care in hospitals, regions, states, and nations depends on precise definitions and the availability of accurate data. The process of matching birth and death certificates is an ideal method for a broad state and national statistical evaluation of mortality because perinatal deaths can be correlated to the hospital or region of origin. The evaluation of perinatal mortality and morbidity should begin, however, at the local hospital. Evaluation of perinatal care should focus on the following goals:

1. Reduce maternal and neonatal morbidity and mortality
2. Evaluate local perinatal programs by identifying problem areas that require improvement and by providing a focus for continuing education of the perinatal health care team
3. Improve local care through a systems approach with special emphasis on validation of the process of risk assessment and management and its effect on the regional approach to perinatal care
4. Provide standard data for hospital-to-hospital comparisons of outcome, evaluations of programs, and studies of comparative epidemiology
5. Document the long-term outcome of perinatal care and practices

Clearly, precise definitions and formulas for the processing of perinatal data, as well as a standard method of evaluation of perinatal care by health care teams centered in the local hospital, are needed to ensure a uniform system of reporting.

This technique for judging the quality of care and detecting problem areas at the local level has limitations that are correctable on a long-term basis. These limitations exist because sufficient data may not be available on official certificates and because at the present time it is difficult for most state data centers to provide local hospitals with timely feedback. Furthermore, as mortality rates have fallen, morbidity evaluation has become increasingly important.

DEFINITIONS

LIVE BIRTH: The complete expulsion or extraction from the mother of a product of human conception, irrespective of the duration of pregnancy, which, after such expulsion or extraction, breathes or shows any other evidence of life, such as beating of the heart, pulsation of the umbilical cord, or definite movement of voluntary muscles whether or not the umbilical cord has been cut or the placenta is attached.

FETAL DEATH: Death prior to the complete expulsion or extraction from the mother of a product of human conception, irrespective of the duration of pregnancy; the death is indicated by the fact that, after such expulsion or extraction, the fetus does not breathe or show any other evidence of life, such as beating of the heart, pulsation of the umbilical cord, or definite movement of voluntary muscles. Fetal death is subdivided according to the timing and mode:

1. *Early fetal death (abortion)*: The explusion or extraction from the mother of a fetus or embryo weighing 500 g or less (about 22 weeks' gestation). This definition excludes induced terminations of pregnancy.

2. *Late fetal death (stillbirth)*: Death prior to expulsion, extraction, or delivery in which the fetal weight is greater than 500 g or, if weight is unknown, the duration of the pregnancy exceeds 22 completed weeks' gestation. When neither birth weight nor gestational age is available, a body length of 25 cm (crown-heel) is considered equivalent to a 500-g weight.

3. *Induced termination of pregnancy*: The deliberate interruption of pregnancy—to produce other than a liveborn neonate or to remove a dead fetus—that does not result in a live birth.

TOTAL BIRTHS: The number of live births plus the number of deaths of fetuses weighing more than 500 g (late fetal deaths).

NEONATAL DEATH: Death of a liveborn neonate before the neonate becomes 28 days old (up to and including 27 days, 23 hours, 59 minutes from the moment of birth). Neonatal deaths may be subdivided, qualified, or defined in other ways for various purposes:

1. *Early neonatal death.* Death of a liveborn neonate during the first 7 days of life (up to and including 6 days, 23 hours, 59 minutes from the moment of birth). These deaths have been described as hebdomadal. For early neonatal deaths, the time of death can be categorized further, using the following intervals or some combination thereof:

Birth to less than 60 completed minutes
1 hour to less than 12 completed hours
12 hours to less than 24 completed hours
24 hours to less than 48 completed hours
48 hours to less than 72 completed hours
72 hours to less than 168 completed hours

2. *Late neonatal death.* Death of a liveborn neonate after 7 completed days (168 hours) but before 28 days of life (27 days, 23 hours, 59 minutes).

Early and late neonatal death statistics are useful for international comparisons. They are terms recommended by the World Health Organization and by the International Federation of Gynecology and Obstetrics.

INFANT DEATH: Any death at any time from birth up to, but not including, 1 year of age.

BIRTH WEIGHT: The weight of a neonate determined immediately after delivery or as soon thereafter as feasible. It should be expressed to the nearest gram. Division into birth weight groups may be required; neonates with birth weights of 1000 g or less may be categorized in 100-, 200-, or 250-g intervals, and neonates with birth weights of 1000–2499 g may be categorized in at least 250-g intervals. Liveborn neonates have traditionally been classified according to weight at birth, and birth weight has been the most commonly used criterion for defining a neonatal population with special risks, as well as for developing uniform national and international vital statistics. Classification based on weight alone equates birth size to fetal age, however, and tends to obscure medically important differences between like-sized neonates of differing gestational age.

GESTATIONAL AGE: The number of completed weeks that have elapsed between the first day of the last normal menstrual period—not the presumed time of conception—and the date of delivery, irrespective of whether the gestation results in a live birth or a fetal death. (See Birth Weight/Gestational Age Classification, Chapter 4.) All neonates can be defined in categories for birth weight-gestational age comparisons: appropriate for gestational age (AGA), small for gestational age (SGA), and large for gestational age (LGA). Graphs and tables of the normal distribution of birth weights over the latter half of gestation are used to classify each birth. Neonates whose birth weights are less than the 10th percentile or greater than the 90th percentile for their population are classified as SGA and LGA, respectively. The interval between death and delivery in cases of fetal death may significantly alter statistics related to gestational age and weight.

CONCEPTIONAL AGE: The number of completed weeks that have elapsed between the time of conception, when accurately known, and the date of delivery. Add 2 weeks to conceptional age to obtain gestational age.

LOW-BIRTH-WEIGHT NEONATE: Any neonate, regardless of gestational age, whose weight at birth is less than 2500 g. A neonate weighing 1500 g or less at birth is considered a very low birth weight neonate.

PRETERM NEONATE: Any neonate whose calculated gestational age from the first day of the last menstrual period is less than 37 completed weeks or 258 completed days.

TERM NEONATE: Any neonate whose gestational age is equal to or greater than 38 weeks but equal to or less than 42 weeks (259–294 days).

POSTTERM NEONATE: Any neonate whose gestational age is greater than 42 weeks (greater than 294 completed days).

MATERNAL DEATH: The death of a woman within 90 days of termination of pregnancy, regardless of duration or site of pregnancy, from any cause related to or aggravated by the pregnancy or its management, but not from accidental or incidental causes. For statistical comparisons with the World Health Organization, it is recommended that two sets of statistics be kept, i.e., maternal deaths within 42 days of termination of pregnancy (WHO), and within 90 days as suggested above for evaluation and comparison within the United States. Even after 90 days, an occasional pregnancy-related maternal death due to conditions such as renal failure or cardiomyopathy may occur and needs to be duly noted.

DIRECT OBSTETRIC DEATH: The death of a woman resulting from obstetric complications of pregnancy, labor, or the puerperium; from interventions, omissions, or incorrect treatment; or from a chain of events resulting from any of these.

INDIRECT OBSTETRIC DEATH: The death of a woman resulting from previously existing disease or disease that developed during pregnancy, labor, or the puerperium that was not due to direct obstetric causes, although the physiologic effects of pregnancy were partially responsible for the death.

It may be useful in a perinatal evaluation to collect data on certain characteristics of the mother, the father, the pregnancy, the care provided, and the newborn. Following is a partial list of categories that should be included in a data base:

1. *Maternal characteristics* include age, gravidity, parity, education, marital status, economic status, race, drug exposure, ingestion of alcohol and smoking, occupational environment, and the presence of concurrent medical-surgical disease.

2. *Paternal characteristics* include age, education, marital status, economic status, race, and the presence of concurrent medical-surgical disease.

3. *Maternal care characteristics* include the date of the initial visit, the number of visits, the type of facility where the visits occurred, antepartum fetal evaluation methods used, the use of monitoring in labor, duration of ruptured membranes, duration of labor, medications administered, and the type of anesthesia for delivery.

4. *Delivery characteristics* include the nature of the labor initiation divided into spontaneous and nonspontaneous (induced) groups. The route of delivery should be designated as vaginal or abdominal, and abdominal deliveries should be further classified as primary or repeat procedures. The fetal presentation, any obstetric complications, and indication for procedures should be noted.

5. *Newborn characteristics* include birth weight, gestational age (method of calculation), sex, Apgar scores at 1 and 5 minutes, head circumference, length, and any other conditions or complications.

STATISTICAL EVALUATION

Uniformity in recording and reporting data is extremely important to facilitate intergroup comparisons. Accuracy and completeness allow for the further subdivision of data into age-specific, weight-specific, and time-specific mortality figures. The following are specific mortality rates that are useful in the evaluation of perinatal care in individual hospitals:

1. Fetal mortality rate is computed by relating deaths of fetuses 500 g and over to total births.

$$\text{Fetal Mortality Rate} = \frac{\text{Fetal Deaths} \geq 500 \text{ g} \times 1000}{\text{Total Number of Births} \geq 500 \text{ g}}$$

2. Neonatal mortality rate is computed by relating deaths during the first 28 days of postnatal life to live births.

$$\text{Neonatal Mortality Rate} = \frac{\text{Neonatal Deaths} < 28 \text{ Days of Age} \times 1000}{\text{Total number of Live Births} \geq 500 \text{ g}}$$

3. Perinatal mortality rate is computed by relating deaths of fetuses 500 g and over plus neonatal deaths during the first 28 days of postnatal life to total births.

$$\text{Perinatal Death Rate} = \frac{\text{Fetal Deaths} \geq 500 \text{ g} + \text{Neonatal Deaths} \times 1000}{\text{Total Number of Births} \geq 500 \text{ g}}$$

Specific perinatal mortality rates may be calculated for any clinical entity, weight, or time period. The denominator must clearly define a population to which the deaths in the numerator belong, and the study period in the numerator and denominator also must coincide. Subsets of a total population can be evaluated, as illustrated in the following examples.

Example 1: Clinical entity, maternal diabetes

$$\text{Perinatal Mortality Rate} = \frac{\begin{array}{c}\text{Fetal Deaths} \geq 500 \text{ g} \\ \text{(Diabetic Mothers)}\end{array} + \begin{array}{c}\text{Neonatal Deaths} \\ \text{(Diabetic Mothers)}\end{array} \times 1000}{\text{Total Births to Diabetic Mothers}}$$

Example 2: Weight-specific neonatal mortality rate

$$\frac{\text{Neonatal Mortality}}{\text{Rate of Neonates}} = \frac{\text{Neonatal Deaths } (1000 < 1500 \text{ g}) \times 1000}{\text{Total Live Births } (1000 < 1500 \text{ g})}$$
$$1000 < 1500 \text{ g}$$

Example 3: Age-specific fetal mortality rate

$$\frac{\text{Fetal Mortality}}{\text{Rate } (32-36 \text{ weeks})} = \frac{\text{Fetal Deaths } (32-36 \text{ weeks}) \times 1000}{\text{Total Births } (32-36 \text{ weeks})}$$

It should be recognized that the fetal death rate plus the neonatal death rate does not equal the perinatal death rate because the denominators are different. The differences, however, are small. These differences may be avoided by expressing each of these as ratios with the same denominator (i.e., live births).

For international comparisons, the following formulas should be used:

$$\frac{\text{Perinatal}}{\text{Mortality}} = \frac{\text{Stillbirths} \geq 1000 \text{ g} + \text{Early Neonatal Deaths} \geq 1000 \text{ g} \times 1000}{\text{Total Births} \geq 1000 \text{ g}}$$
$$\text{Rate}$$

$$\frac{\text{Early Neonatal}}{\text{Mortality Rate}} = \frac{\text{Early Neonatal Deaths} \geq 1000 \text{ g at Birth} \times 1000}{\text{Live Births} \geq 1000 \text{ g}}$$

$$\frac{\text{Fetal Mortality}}{\text{Rate}} = \frac{\text{Stillbirths} \geq 1000 \text{ g} \times 1000}{\text{Total Births} \geq 1000 \text{ g}}$$

Figure 9-1 presents a schematic representation of the categories of pregnancy outcome.

LOCAL HOSPITAL EVALUATION

The major concern of the practicing physician and the local hospital is to provide the best quality care for patients. Regional and national statistics rarely pinpoint local problems; the most meaningful evaluation originates at the local hospital. The process of evaluation at the local level should be simple in design, should involve minimal paperwork and maximal visibility, and should provide for input from all members of the health care team. The following suggestions meet these criteria and can be easily adapted and expanded as local expertise in evaluation is gained; there is no single solution to the problem of local evaluation.

A single, multicopy obstetric and neonatal discharge summary is designed to provide complete information for maternal and neonatal charts, for the obstetrician, for the pediatrician, and for a predetermined hospital body charged with concurrent review of care. In addition, a simple monthly publication of statistics, which can be easily tabulated from the delivery and nursery logs, should be prominently displayed in obstetric and newborn units. Deaths should be recorded on a separate document, listing date, hospital unit number, name, birth weight, and presumptive cause of death. This allows for easy identification and regular local peer review. Periodically (perhaps 1/100–150 deliveries), the health care team should meet to review summaries and address key questions regarding each death. The team may also focus on specific procedures or diagnoses. Yearly review by an outside consultant can provide further critical evaluation as well as important learning experiences for all members of the health care team. Trends in care can easily be documented by simple tabulation, graphic illustration, and display of several years of data.

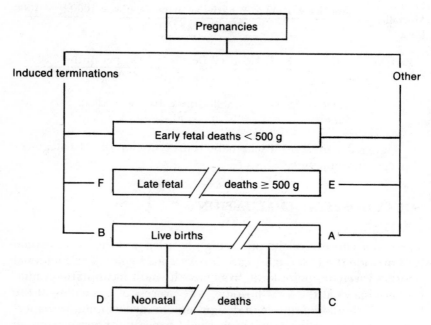

Fig. 9-1. *Algorithm for evaluation of pregnancy outcomes. For some purposes of local evaluation, D and F may be omitted from the definition of perinatal mortality. Live births = A + B; neonatal deaths = C + D; fetal deaths = E + F; total births = A + B + E + F;*

$$perinatal\ mortality\ rate = \frac{C + D + E + F}{A + B + E + F} \times 1000$$

chapter # 10
Special Considerations

Antenatal Detection of Genetic Disorders

Antenatal detection of genetic disorders has become an accepted part of medical care for mother and child. Collaborative studies have verified the reliability of the approach, and consensus statements have been published. Symposia and textbooks have reviewed in detail current indications and future directions; this information is summarized to present the current status of antenatal diagnosis as it relates to obstetric and pediatric practice.

IDENTIFICATION OF COUPLES AT INCREASED RISK FOR GENETIC DISORDERS

Couples at increased risk for bearing genetically abnormal offspring usually are identified on the basis of advanced parental age or the presence of an anomaly in the prospective father or mother, their previous offspring, or a near relative. Repetitive abortions or stillbirths also constitute grounds for investigation. In addition, certain autosomal recessive diseases are sufficiently common to warrant screening for heterozygosity. For example, Ashkenazim Jews should be screened to identify individuals heterozygous for Tay-Sachs disease.

To facilitate identification of such couples, brief questionnaires are available. Couples at increased risk may or may not need formal genetic consultation. Sometimes the problem is relatively uncomplicated. For example, the relationship between advanced maternal age and chromosomal abnormalities is well-known (Table 10–1) and readily communicated by the primary physician. In other cases, complexities may justify referral. Whatever the situation, counseling is oblig-

Table 10-1. Risk of Having a Liveborn Child with Down's Syndrome by 1-Year Maternal Age Intervals from 20–49 Years

Maternal age	Risk of Down's syndrome
20	1/1923
21	1/1695
22	1/1538
23	1/1408
24	1/1299
25	1/1205
26	1/1124
27	1/1053
28	1/990
29	1/935
30	1/885
31	1/826
32	1/725
33	1/592
34	1/465
35	1/365
36	1/287
37	1/225
38	1/177
39	1/139
40	1/109
41	1/85
42	1/67
43	1/53
44	1/41
45	1/32
46	1/25
47	1/20
48	1/16
49	1/12

(Data from Hook EB, Chamber GM: Estimated rates of Down's syndrome in live births by 1-year maternal age intervals for mothers aged 20–49 in a New York state study—Implications of the risk figures for genetic counseling and cost-benefit analysis of prenatal diagnosis programs. Birth Defects 13:124, 1977)

atory prior to antenatal diagnostic studies. Every couple should be informed of their increased risk for fetal abnormalities, the availability of antenatal diagnosis, and the prognosis for liveborn affected off-spring. Most counselors agree that their function is not to dictate a particular course but to provide information that will allow couples to make informed decisions.

Genetic services have been receiving more attention, and attempts are being made to structure and certify individual responsibilities. Historically, pediatricians and obstetricians have done much of the clinical and investigative work. Nurses have emerged as counselors and program coordinators. Other professionals have also made important contributions to clinical human genetics. These activities will continue; a certification program that identifies different roles, such as physician subspecialist or genetic associate, is in place.

Regional genetic programs are already functioning in some areas. Close coordination, perhaps integration, of programmatic and individual clinical activity involving genetic and perinatal concerns is necessary. Genetic counseling will probably become an increasingly important part of regional perinatal program activity.

Relatively uncomplicated antenatal genetic detection problems can be managed by the primary physician—obstetrician or pediatrician—individually or in a structured relationship with a trained nurse-clinician, genetic associate, or other geneticist. If the condition is complicated, a medical geneticist should be involved.

TECHNICAL CONSIDERATIONS

Amniocentesis

Antenatal assessment for genetic disorders usually requires amniocentesis. Transabdominal amniocentesis for genetic purposes should be performed before 20 weeks of pregnancy, preferably in the 16th week. It is recommended that ultrasonography be performed prior to amniocentesis in order to determine fetal maturity, localize the placenta, and exclude multiple gestations. A small gauge spinal needle is placed transabdominally to aspirate 20–35 ml amniotic fluid. An experienced obstetrician will obtain the required volume of fluid on the initial attempt in at least 95% of cases. Cultures usually require 3–4 weeks, and cytogenetic and biochemical analysis are almost always accurate (99%).

Amniocentesis is not without some risk for mother and fetus. Although significant maternal injury virtually never occurs, abortion sometimes follows the procedure. Unexplained differences in the abortion rates have been observed in several collaborative studies, all involving centers in which amniocenteses were performed in large numbers by relatively few, skilled individuals; however, the additional risk for abortion secondary to transabdominal amniocentesis is apparently not greater than 0.5%–1%. Severe injury to the surviving fetus is extremely rare.

Fetoscopy

Use of fetoscopy for visualization of the fetus or for fetal blood sampling has been feasible for several years, and considerable experience has been gathered at selected centers. Fetoscopy requires considerably more experience than does amniocentesis and thus is available in only a few centers. Application of this technology is limited because the abortion risk after midtrimester fetoscopy and fetal blood sampling is increased by about 5%. In addition, the risk for premature delivery appears to be increased after fetoscopy.

Laboratory Studies

It may be necessary for physicians to communicate with laboratory personnel in order to ensure proper referral of patients, and collection and handling of specimens. Physicians should be aware that many laboratories perform cytogenetic (chromosome) analyses, but relatively few perform certain metabolic tests. Thus, it may be necessary to ship amniotic fluid or cultured cells to regional or national centers. Laboratories that process amniotic fluid specimens should utilize accepted methods of quality control to minimize culture failures and diagnostic errors.

ACCEPTED INDICATIONS

Consideration of both potential benefits and risks has resulted in the following accepted indications for intrauterine monitoring:

1. Cytogenetic indications
   a. Advanced maternal age (35 years or older at expected time of delivery)
   b. Previous offspring with a chromosomal aberration, particularly autosomal trisomy
   c. Chromosomal abnormality in either parent, particularly a translocation
   d. Determination of fetal sex when a serious X-linked condition for which specific intrauterine diagnosis is not available may be present
2. Inborn errors of metabolism detectable in amniotic fluid or cultured amniotic fluid cells
3. Neural tube defects
4. Hemoglobinopathies (The antenatal diagnosis of hemoglobinopathies remains in the developmental stage. Advances in molecular genetics, specifically, application of restriction enzymes and deoxyribonucleic acid (DNA) probes, permit detection of α-thalassemia, sickle cell anemia, and often β-thalassemia in cultured amniotic fluid fibroblasts solely on the basis of DNA sequence.)

ADDITIONAL INDICATIONS AND FUTURE DIRECTIONS

Antenatal cytogenetic studies may be appropriate in many other circumstances, depending on preferences of patients and availability of scientific expertise. It is unrealistic to expect primary physicians to be familiar with all the latest genetic advances. Practitioners should therefore seek consultations with specialists in antenatal diagnosis.

Visualization of the fetus by ultrasonography, roentgenography, and fetoscopy is under active investigation. Diagnosis of certain birth defects may be feasible with each of these methods. In particular, more advanced ultrasonography has been used to evaluate hydrocephalus, neural tube defects, renal abnormalities, skeletal abnormalities, cardiac anomalies, and other defects. Highly skilled ultrasonographers have been able to predict fetal outcomes correctly on the basis of midtrimester studies, although neither sensitivity nor specificity is well defined. Ultrasonography plays an essential adjunctive role in dating pregnancies and excluding multiple gestations whenever antenatal studies are planned.

Fetoscopic blood sampling is utilized for the diagnosis of hemoglobinopathies, hemophilia, and other disorders. Moreover, fetoscopic skin biopsies have been used to diagnose certain congenital skin disorders that have an unknown metabolic basis. The relatively high risks of fetoscopy have spurred attempts to detect hemoglobinopathies in utero by safer techniques. In the future, molecular techniques should permit midtrimester diagnosis of many genetic disorders that are not currently detectable. However, DNA studies are not widely available and at present should be performed only under the aegis of clinical investigation.

In addition to more direct methods for antenatal diagnosis, the presence or absence of mutant genes can sometimes be inferred by analysis of a closely linked polymorphic locus (linkage analysis). For example, linkage between human leukocyte antigen (HLA) and 21-hydroxylase deficiency (adrenal hyperplasia) permits diagnosis of the latter. Linkage analysis should become more useful as more genes are localized to specific chromosomes and more DNA polymorphisms are identified.

Clinical Considerations in the Use of Oxygen

Hazards associated with the administration of oxygen therapy to prematurely born neonates have been recognized for almost three decades. Prolonged use of supplemental oxygen concentrations in neonates of very low birth weight, i.e., those who weigh less than 1500 g, has been associated with an increased incidence of retrolental fibroplasia (RLF), which is sometimes referred to as retinopathy of prematurity. No such association with short-term hyperoxia has been demonstrated, however. It is noteworthy that when the practice was to restrict oxygen use, the incidence of RLF decreased; however, the mortality rate of neonates with hyaline membrane disease increased, as did the number of neonates surviving with spastic diplegia and other neurologic disorders.

Although it appears that ischemia of the retina, particularly of the immature retina, may initiate the vasoproliferative process leading to RLF, many factors other than simple hyperoxia can play an important role in the pathogenesis of RLF. Apnea, asphyxia, sepsis, nutritional deficiencies, numerous and frequent blood transfusions, prolonged periods of oxygen therapy, and long periods of ventilatory support, especially in association with hypercarbia and hypoxia, have all been related to RLF.

Attempts to correlate the level of the partial pressure of oxygen in blood (PaO_2) with the development of RLF have thus far been unsuccessful. RLF has occurred in neonates who have never received supplemental oxygen, in neonates with cyanotic congenital heart disease whose PaO_2 level could not have been greater than 50 mm Hg, and in full-term neonates. Neonates also have developed severe changes of RLF in one eye with little, if any, abnormality in the other eye. Conversely, many small premature neonates have had periods of sustained hyperoxia without developing RLF. Neonates who have been monitored continuously with skin surface electrodes have developed RLF, even when scrupulous attempts have been made to maintain the PaO_2 levels within an accepted range.

MANAGEMENT

No criteria have as yet been established to guarantee the safe use of oxygen in the management of newborns with various cardiopulmonary abnormalities. Factors that may have contributed in part to this problem involve (1) previous inability to measure PaO_2 levels continuously over long periods of time in the very low-birth-weight neonates and (2) the possibility of shunting of blood from right to left in those neonates. Because of biologic variations, as well as the aforementioned factors and other unknown causes, concentrations of oxygen that may be safe for one newborn may not be safe for another. Supplemental oxygen should be used with caution; it is prudent to attempt to maintain the neonate's PaO_2 within the range of that of normal newborns—50–100 mm Hg. In addition to avoiding hyperoxia, it is equally important to avoid periods of hypoxia and compromised perfusion, which also may lead to retinal ischemia and aberrant proliferation of the immature retinal vessels. In very small and very sick neonates, these conditions are often unavoidable, despite all precautions.

Skin color cannot be used to estimate PaO_2 levels reliably. Measurements of the partial pressure of oxygen in arterial blood are necessary to manage the neonate optimally.

MONITORING TECHNIQUES

With the development of transcutaneous oxygen electrodes, the skin surface PO_2 level can be measured continuously and for relatively long periods. Although these electrodes have made it possible to maintain the neonate's PaO_2 level in a more "normal" range, they may not accurately reflect the PaO_2 level, especially in states of poor perfusion, hypovolemia, or shock.

It is important to evaluate skin perfusion carefully. In addition, the electrodes have to be checked frequently to ensure that they are indeed reflecting the neonate's PaO_2 level. This is a simple procedure when the neonate has an in-dwelling arterial catheter, but it becomes more difficult when catheters or arterial lines are no longer in place. Intermittent arterial punctures have been used to verify the validity of the skin surface electrode measurements, but performing this on neonates weighing less than 1000 g is extremely difficult and often impossible. If the neonate cries or becomes apneic, the values from the arterial blood gas analysis are difficult to interpret. It is questionable whether this is a reliable indicator of the neonate's PaO_2 level at rest. The use of transcutaneous oxygen electrodes and interpretation of their measurements need additional evaluation.

CONCLUSIONS AND RECOMMENDATIONS

The current state of knowledge warrants the following conclusions:

1. RLF is a condition that is not currently preventable in some neo-

nates, especially those of very low birth weight and those who require supplemental oxygen for prolonged periods, in spite of meticulous monitoring and care.

2. Many factors other than simple hyperoxia can be important in the pathogenesis of RLF in any given patient.

3. Transient elevations in PaO_2 cannot be implicated with confidence as the proximate cause of RLF.

4. No standards have as yet been established to guarantee the safe use of oxygen in neonates.

Taking into account the current, but incomplete, understanding of the effects of oxygen administration and its association with the occurrence of RLF, the following recommendations can be made:

1. No neonate should receive supplemental oxygen unless there is a specific indication for its use, such as cyanosis or respiratory distress.

2. When a neonate whose gestational age is 36 weeks or less requires supplemental oxygen, the concentration of inspired oxygen should be regulated soon after its initiation by measuring arterial oxygen tension or by following the neonate's skin surface PaO_2 level. If the place of birth has no facilities for measuring arterial oxygen tension, the prematurely born neonate who requires oxygen for any reason should be given oxygen in concentrations just sufficient to abolish cyanosis. The neonate should be moved as soon as possible to a center capable of measuring arterial oxygen tension levels.

3. When a neonate whose gestational age is greater than 36 weeks requires supplemental oxygen, the neonate should be given oxygen initially in concentrations great enough to abolish cyanosis. Those who require oxygen for more than a few hours should be transferred to a center where arterial oxygen tension can be measured and diagnostic studies and therapeutic measures can be initiated.

4. When supplemental oxygen is given to the premature neonate, an attempt should be made to maintain the PaO_2 at a level not greater than 100 mm Hg, preferably between 50–90 mm Hg. Even with careful monitoring, the PaO_2 may fluctuate excessively beyond this range, especially in neonates with cardiopulmonary disease. If hyperoxia occurs, the inspired oxygen concentration should be lowered gradually in order to prevent a rapid fall in the PaO_2 level. It may be prudent to maintain a neonate's PaO_2

level over 100 mm Hg when attempts to lower the concentration of inspired oxygen result in a dramatic fall of the neonate's PaO_2 to dangerously low levels. The concurrent risk of RLF may be unavoidable during such periods. This is especially true of neonates with pulmonary hypertension. Even when the inspired oxygen concentration is lowered gradually and with caution, the neonate may respond so dramatically that hypoxemia and hypercarbia result. When the PaO_2 level falls rapidly in such situations, it is frequently difficult, if not impossible, to restabilize the neonate. The neonate's record should reflect the physician's decision, which is based on clinical judgment of the situation, and the communication to the parents of this decision and its risks.*

5. Although 100% oxygen is used frequently to resuscitate a hypoxic or asphyxiated neonate, the use of these high concentrations of oxygen in the postresuscitation and stabilization periods should be monitored in conjunction with the measurement of the neonate's PaO_2 levels. This is also important during the transport of neonates to intensive care nurseries. Transcutaneous monitoring of oxygen may be helpful in these situations.

6. When arterial blood cannot be sampled readily or when transcutaneous oxygen monitoring is unavailable or found to be unreliable for a specific patient, arterialized capillary samples have been used to monitor arterial oxygen. Unfortunately, while these samples seem to correlate well when the PaO_2 level is less than 50 mm Hg, they do not correlate well when the PaO_2 level is greater than 50 mm Hg. Even when the arterialized capillary sample is the only available method to monitor arterial oxygen, the values must be interpreted with caution.

7. When any neonate is in an oxygen-enriched environment, the concentration of oxygen in the environment should be recorded every hour and monitored carefully with an oxygen analyzer. The setting of a reliable oxygen-air mixture should be noted and recorded at least every hour. The analyzer and the oxygen-air mixture should be calibrated and recorded every 8 hours with both room air and 100% oxygen. Records of these measurements should be kept in addition to those of the PaO_2 or the neonate's skin surface PaO_2 level.

---

*These recommendations differ significantly from those in *Standards and Recommendations for Hospital Care of Newborn Infants*, 6 ed, published in 1977 by AAP.

8. Except in an emergency, oxygen and compressed air should be humidified and warmed before administration to a neonate.

9. Careful monitoring of pH, $Paco_2$ and blood pressure levels are also recommended. Sustained periods of hypercarbia and hypotension should be avoided if at all possible.

10. An individual experienced in neonatal opthalmology and indirect opthalmoscopy should dilate and examine the retinas of those prematurely born neonates treated with oxygen when they are 6–8 weeks of age. If the neonate is discharged from the hospital prior to that time, arrangements should be made for follow-up evaluation. The exact timing of the examinations may vary from institution to institution and from opthalmologist to opthalmologist; these are suggested guidelines. These examinations serve to identify those patients who have RLF. If active disease is observed, more frequent examinations are indicated until the disease has reached a quiescent stage. Yearly examinations are recommended for those who have had evidence of active disease.

11. There is no clear evidence that therapy to treat RLF, once it has developed, is effective. Recent controlled studies have demonstrated that the prophylactic administration of 50–100 mg/kg/day vitamin E to neonates weighing 1500 g or less may reduce the severity, but not the incidence of RLF. However, the information about toxicity of vitamin E is insufficient at present to allow a recommendation for the routine prophylactic use of this agent in all neonates weighing less than 1500 g.

Hyperbilirubinemia

The diagnosis of kernicterus is occasionally established at autopsy, but the relationship between serum bilirubin levels below 20 mg/dl (342 μmol/liter)* and kernicterus in full-term and low-birth-weight neonates is not clear. Subtle neurodevelopmental impairment may be associated with hyperbilirubinemia in some neonates. The incidence of such impairment is not known, nor is it known at what bilirubin level below 20 mg/dl (342 μmol/liter) or under what other circumstances the risk of brain damage exceeds the risk of treatment. There are no simple solutions in the management of jaundiced neonates.

BILIRUBIN TOXICITY

A direct association between severe, unconjugated hyperbilirubinemia and kernicterus has been demonstrated in neonates with erythroblastosis fetalis. Neonates who die with kernicterus demonstrate yellowish discoloration of the brain with specific yellow staining of the nuclear areas. Survivors often manifest serious neurologic sequelae, particularly the athetoid form of cerebral palsy, hearing loss, paralysis of upward gaze, and dental dysplasia. Observations made some 30 years ago suggested that, in full-term neonates with erythroblastosis fetalis, kernicterus was very unlikely to occur if serum bilirubin concentrations were kept below 20 mg/dl (342 μmol/liter); subsequent experience in the care of such neonates has justified these conclusions. In some studies, an association has been found between an increase in bilirubin levels during the neonatal period and poor developmental outcome.

With increasing emphasis on neonatal intensive care, much concern has been expressed regarding the risk of kernicterus in sick, low-birth-weight neonates. These concerns result from case reports documenting the presence of kernicterus at autopsy in premature neonates whose bilirubin levels did not exceed 10 mg/dl (171 μmol/liter). As a result, published guidelines for the management of jaundice in such neonates suggest early phototherapy and exchange transfusion at bilirubin levels as low as 10 mg/dl (171 μmol/liter).

It has been assumed that if kernicterus can be documented (at autopsy) at very low bilirubin levels, then perhaps bilirubin-related brain damage is occurring in some surviving neonates whose serum bilirubin concentrations did not exceed 10 mg/dl (171 μmol/liter).

---

*1 mg/dl = 17.1 μmol/liter.

However, several studies of low-birth-weight neonates have been unable to identify any relationship between bilirubin levels and later neurodevelopmental handicap, particularly if serum bilirubin levels did not exceed 20 mg/dl (342 μmol/liter). The number of patients in these studies might not have been large enough, however, to detect an effect, if one existed. Nevertheless, two recent studies of low-birth-weight neonates failed to identify the serum bilirubin level as a risk factor for kernicterus. In addition, risk factors such as sepsis, hypothermia, asphyxia, acidosis, hypercarbia, hypoxia, hypoglycemia, and hypoalbuminemia, when present, did not increase significantly the risk of kernicterus at a given level of serum bilirubin. In neither of these studies could any single factor or combination of factors (including serum bilirubin concentrations) be associated with an increased risk for kernicterus.

These studies underscore the extreme complexity of attempting to correlate levels of serum bilirubin and subsequent neurologic status. Furthermore, it must be emphasized that the finding of an association between poor intellectual outcome and certain bilirubin levels in a large group of neonates, although suggestive, does not alone provide incontrovertible evidence of a cause-and-effect relationship. When large population groups are studied, minor differences in outcome may become statistically significant, but how this information can be applied rationally to the management of the individual neonate with jaundice is, as yet, undetermined. No properly designed clinical studies (i.e., clinical experiments) have been performed that permit a definition of bilirubin levels at which the risk of kernicterus exceeds the risk of exchange transfusion in neonates. Nevertheless, there is legitimate concern that subtle neurodevelopmental impairment may represent part of a continuum of neurologic damage associated with hyperbilirubinemia.

It has been widely believed that bilirubin must be "free," or unbound to albumin, in order to cross the blood-brain barrier. An increase in free bilirubin in the presence of normal or low total serum bilirubin levels is the explanation most frequently advanced for the lack of correlation between total serum bilirubin levels and autopsy evidence of kernicterus in low-birth-weight neonates. Although there is evidence from animal studies to support this theory, it has not been tested critically in neonates. Furthermore, the correlation between measured free bilirubin levels* and the presence of kernicterus at autopsy is not

---

*It is questionable whether free bilirubin actually can be measured and the methodology is fraught with difficulties. A better term for clinical use is *apparent unbound bilirubin concentration*.

consistent. Finally, recent animal studies have provided direct proof that, when the blood-brain barrier is disrupted, albumin-bound bilirubin will enter the brain. Thus, one possible explanation for the lack of correlation between total (or free) bilirubin levels and the development of kernicterus is an alteration in the permeability of the blood-brain barrier.

The kernicterus reported in premature neonates with very low bilirubin levels has been documented only at autopsy. Whether such neonates would have suffered neurologic damage, had they recovered, is unknown. In addition, finding of bilirubin staining at autopsy in these neonates might be secondary to prior, nonspecific damage rather than an indication of bilirubin toxicity.

CLINICAL MANAGEMENT OF THE JAUNDICED NEONATE

If there is any evidence that the jaundice is not physiologic, it should be investigated prior to the initiation of treatment. When carefully reviewed, the data from numerous studies of bilirubin toxicity are so complex they permit almost no rational conclusions regarding the therapeutic approach to these neonates. No single test of albumin binding of bilirubin has been shown to be sufficiently reliable to be recommended for clinical use, nor have such tests been shown to be more helpful than measurements of indirect serum bilirubin in the prevention of kernicterus. The current use of these tests should be restricted to properly designed studies.

Numerous guidelines on the management of jaundiced neonates have been published, but they have not been tested experimentally. Over the past two decades, clinical observations (not experiments) in full-term neonates with hemolytic disease of the newborn have confirmed that the occurrence of clinical kernicterus is highly unlikely if serum unconjugated bilirubin levels are kept below 20 mg/dl (342 μmol/liter). There are no properly designed studies, however, or even observational data in low-birth-weight neonates (or full-term neonates without hemolytic disease) that permit scientific recommendations to be made regarding the treatment of such neonates with serum bilirubin levels below 20 mg/dl (342 μmol/liter).

Many physicians currently use published guidelines and are aggressive in their treatment of jaundice in low-birth-weight neonates, initiating phototherapy early and performing exchange transfusions in certain neonates with very low bilirubin levels (<10 mg/dl). Nevertheless, it must be recognized that this will not prevent kernicterus consistently. Some pediatricians may prefer to adopt a more conservative therapeutic stance and allow serum bilirubin levels to approach 15–20 mg/dl (257–342 μmol/liter), even in low-birth-weight neonates, before considering exchange transfusion. At present, both of these approaches to treatment must be considered acceptable. In either case, the finding of low bilirubin kernicterus at autopsy in certain low-birth-weight neonates cannot necessarily be interpreted as a therapeutic failure. Like retrolental fibroplasia, kernicterus is a condition that, in certain neonates, is essentially unpreventable.

Although there is some evidence of an association between hyperbilirubinemia and neurodevelopmental handicap less severe than classical kernicterus, it has not been established that this represents a cause-and-effect relationship. Furthermore, there is no information presently available to suggest that treating mild jaundice will prevent such handicap.

Hemolytic Disease

In the presence of hemolytic disease, the indications for the first exchange transfusion should be based on serial determinations of the serum bilirubin level and not on cord blood levels of hemoglobin and bilirubin (unless the neonate is hydropic or has a life-threatening anemia). Some physicians also consider the rate of rise of serum bilirubin levels. A useful "rule of thumb" for indicating that the bilirubin level is likely to reach 20 mg/dl (342 μmol/liter) is a serum bilirubin level of 10 mg/dl (171 μmol/liter) by 24 hours or 15 mg/dl (257 μmol/liter) by 48 hours in spite of phototherapy. Women who are likely to deliver severely affected, hydropic neonates should be managed exclusively in perinatal centers capable of the full range of obstetric and neonatal intensive care.

Breast-Feeding and Jaundice

Many pediatricians have had the impression that breast-fed neonates have higher serum bilirubin levels during the first week of life than bottle-fed neonates. This concept of jaundice associated with breast-feeding (which must be distinguished from true breast milk jaundice) rests, for the moment, on a body of data that is by no means secure. The composite data from eight recent studies reveal that on days 3–6 breast-fed babies have serum bilirubin levels that are 0.8 mg/dl (14 μmol/liter) higher than those found in bottle-fed babies. These differences are not clinically important.

There is no evidence that weight loss associated with breast-feeding is in any way related to serum bilirubin levels, nor is there any information to suggest that providing supplemental water or formula to such neonates will affect serum bilirubin levels. In addition, when an elevated indirect serum bilirubin level is due to some pathologic cause, there is no reason to interdict breast-feeding. The finding of an association between breast-feeding and increased levels of serum bilirubin does not imply a causal relationship.

Breast Milk Jaundice

About 1%–2% of breast-fed babies develop the syndrome of breast milk jaundice. The serum bilirubin concentration rises progressively from about the fourth day of life and reaches a maximum level of unconjugated bilirubin of 10–30 mg/dl (171–513 μmol/liter) by 10–15 days of life. If breast-feeding continues, elevated levels may persist for 4–10 days, then decline slowly, and reach normal values by 3–12 weeks of age. However, if breast-feeding is interrupted at any stage, there is a prompt decline in serum bilirubin levels within 48 hours. With the resumption of nursing, the bilirubin concentration may rise 1–3 mg/dl (17–51 μmol/liter), but it does not reach the previous level. There is no evidence of hemolysis, and the results of liver function studies are normal.

Although no cases of overt bilirubin encephalopathy related to breast milk jaundice have been reported, there have been no prospective studies of either term or preterm neonates with this condition. Furthermore, there is no reason to believe that significant elevations of serum bilirubin in the breast-fed neonate represent less of a threat than do similar elevations in the bottle-fed neonate. When the bilirubin concentration in breast-fed neonates is rising and it appears that it will reach 20 mg/dl (342 μmol/liter), it is suggested that nursing be interrupted for 48 hours. This is almost invariably followed by a prompt decline in bilirubin levels, and nursing can then be resumed.

Positive and enthusiastic support should be provided to these nursing mothers, and they should be encouraged to maintain lactation using a breast pump or manual expression during the period of interrupted nursing. They should also be reassured that there is nothing wrong with them or their milk. This approach rarely results in permanent cessation of nursing and does not affect the mother's subsequent ability to nurse her neonate. In fact, the usual rapid decline in bilirubin that occurs with the interruption of nursing is reassuring and allows the mother to resume her nursing without having to be concerned about bilirubin levels and further blood tests.

Phototherapy

Used extensively throughout the world, phototherapy is an effective means of reducing serum bilirubin concentrations. It appears to be more effective than exchange transfusion in achieving prolonged reduction of bilirubin levels in neonates with nonhemolytic jaundice. Exchange transfusion, however, remains the only certain way of lowering serum bilirubin rapidly. Phototherapy modifies the course of hyperbilirubinemia in ABO and Rh hemolytic disease and reduces, but does not eliminate, the need for exchange transfusion. Whether this is beneficial to neonates treated in this fashion is unknown.

Characteristics of Light Source and the Dose-Response Relationship

Various types of fluorescent light as well as a quartz halide light have been used for phototherapy. A minimum irradiance of 4 $\mu W/cm^2/nm$ in the blue spectrum (as measured by a photometer) appears to be necessary for effective phototherapy. The response increases concurrently with increasing dose until a saturation point is reached (about 10–12 $\mu W/cm^2/nm$). Because different instruments provide readouts in different units, caution should be exercised in interpreting measurements from photometers. Blue lights are most effective, presumably because they have an energy output near the maximal absorption peak of bilirubin. Unfortunately, such lights produce undesirable color changes in the neonates and may produce discomfort and vertigo in the nursery staff. A combination of four special blue lamps placed in the center of the phototherapy unit with two daylight lamps on either side has been found to provide excellent irradiance without producing significant discomfort to personnel.

Indications for Phototherapy

Phototherapy is indicated when serum bilirubin levels are rising and approach the level at which exchange transfusion is likely to be considered. A suggested guideline is to decide on the level at which exchange transfusion will be performed and to initiate phototherapy at a serum bilirubin concentration 5 mg/dl below that point, although in the presence of hemolytic disease, it might be appropriate to start phototherapy earlier (see Hemolytic Disease, this chapter). In many nurseries phototherapy is used at much lower bilirubin levels, particularly in very small neonates. At present, there is no evidence to show that this has been either helpful or harmful. If the diagnosis is breast milk jaundice, it is more effective to interrupt nursing temporarily than to initiate phototherapy.

Toxicity

As far as can be determined, the risk of toxicity with phototherapy is extremely low. No overt toxicity has been identified in the human neonate. Nevertheless, phototherapy has many biologic effects and long-term follow-up studies of such neonates are still needed. Because animal experiments have documented retinal damage from phototherapy, it is recommended that the neonate's eyes be covered with opaque patches during phototherapy. These patches can become displaced and obstruct the nares, however, causing apnea and even asphyxia. Constant supervision is necessary to avoid this potential hazard.

Lamp Life

The life of a lamp varies widely in different circumstances and with different lamps. Overheating in the light chamber produces deterioration of the phosphors and shortens lamp life, but, with adequate cooling, lamp life is usually several thousand hours. To ensure lamp effectiveness, however, it is useful to measure the energy output with a photometer.

Conclusions

The information reviewed in this section is the best current appraisal of the existing data and its application to the care of the jaundiced infant, as summarized in the following conclusions:

1. Observations over the past two decades have confirmed that clinical kernicterus is very unlikely to occur in full-term neonates with erythroblastosis fetalis if serum bilirubin concentrations are kept below 20 mg/dl (342 μmol/liter).

2. There are no data in the form of clinical observations in properly designed studies that permit scientific recommendations to be made regarding the use of exchange transfusions in low-birth-weight neonates with serum bilirubin levels below 20 mg/dl (342 μmol/liter) for the prevention of kernicterus.

3. Even aggressive management of jaundice in the low-birth-weight neonate, including early phototherapy and exchange transfusions in certain neonates with very low bilirubin levels (less than 10 mg/dl), will not consistently prevent kernicterus.

4. The finding of kernicterus at autopsy in certain low-birth-weight neonates whose bilirubin levels have been low cannot necessarily be interpreted as a therapeutic failure.

5. Although there is some evidence of an association between hyperbilirubinemia and neurodevelopmental handicap less severe than classical kernicterus, it has not been established that this is a cause-and-effect relationship. There are no data to suggest that treating mild jaundice prevents the handicap.

6. Like retrolental fibroplasia, kernicterus is a condition that, in certain neonates, is essentially unpreventable by current practice.

Thermal Regulation

The importance of maintaining the core temperature of a neonate within the range of 36°–37.5° C is well-known. Normally, thermoregulatory control mechanisms maintain a balance between heat production and heat loss so that body temperature remains constant at about 37° C. The high surface/mass ratio of the newborn, especially the low-birth-weight newborn, is particularly suited for the emission of heat, however. External heat or cold stress readily overrides the thermoregulatory control system of the sick low-birth-weight neonate with serious, even lethal, consequences.

After delivery, a thermal environment that is optimal for the neonate should be maintained. This has been assumed to be the range of ambient temperature within which the neonate's oxygen consumption (an indirect measurement of heat production) and thermoregulatory water loss are at a minimum and normal body temperature is maintained. However, the thermoneutral zone (i.e., the range of ambient temperature within which metabolic rate is at a minimum and temperature regulation is achieved by nonevaporative physical processes alone) of the naked newborn is fairly narrow and cannot be measured routinely. There is also considerable variation in basal metabolism among neonates. Thus, it is difficult to predict accurately the thermal environment in which an individual neonate's rate of oxygen consumption will be minimal. In addition, metabolic rate is related to the neonate's body size, postnatal age, and clinical status, as well as to physical factors in the nursery that cannot be controlled completely. At best, the suggested temperature range for the thermoneutral zone for neonates in the nursery is only an approximate prediction of the thermal conditions most likely to maintain normal body temperature at minimal metabolic cost to the neonates.

The site selected for taking a neonate's temperature should be recorded and used consistently in making serial measurements. Moreover, because of inconsistencies in the accuracy of clinical thermometers, the same thermometer (whether glass or electronic) should be used for serial measurements made in an individual neonate. Consistency in the technique of measurement also facilitates interpretation of recorded fluctuations in temperature.

Normal axillary and rectal temperatures range from 36.5°–37.5° C. The axillary temperature is taken by placing a clinical thermometer deep in the axilla while the arm is held gently, but firmly, against the chest for 3 minutes. Rectal temperatures generally should not be taken. Deep body temperature can be measured in the rectum, esophagus, or auditory canal by means of an appropriate flexible thermometer.

The body temperature of vigorous term neonates should be determined when they are admitted to the nursery and at no less than 4-hour intervals until it is in the normal range and stable. Thereafter, temperature should be determined and recorded, preferably, on each 8-hour shift. Body temperature of low-birth-weight neonates should be monitored continuously by thermistors or be determined at intervals of 1–3 hours. Normal skin temperature, as measured by a thermistor taped to the anterior abdominal wall, is 36°–36.5° C.

DELIVERY ROOM CARE

Under usual delivery room conditions, it is not possible to prevent completely the losses of body heat that follow birth. Most neonates inevitably suffer some cold stress at the time of delivery because of large radiant, convective, and evaporative heat losses from their warm, wet skin. Their skin temperature may fall precipitously by 0.3° C/minute; rectal temperature decreases more slowly. Most contemporary delivery rooms are air-conditioned; room temperature may have to be adjusted in consideration of the neonate.

In low-birth-weight neonates, the surface/mass ratio is exaggerated; their tissues exhibit increased thermal conductivity, and heat loss per unit of surface area is enhanced. Asphyxia, anesthesia, maternal sedation, infection, and birth injury may all have adverse effects on thermal stability of the newborn.

Even healthy, term neonates have a limited thermogenic response to a cool environment over the first 12 hours of life, and heat loss should be minimized during this period. Neonates should not be bathed or washed until thermal stability is ensured. The following steps can reduce heat loss after birth:

1. Dry the neonate completely with prewarmed towels. The head and face, which constitute a large surface area, are particularly important.

2. Use a radiant heater above the neonate and a warming mattress to create a heat-gaining environment.

3. Wrap the neonate with a dry, warm blanket, an aluminum swaddler, or a transparent plastic bag to reduce heat loss.

4. Use a radiant heat source positioned over the mother and neonate to prevent cooling of neonates kept with their mothers in the delivery room.

THERMAL ENVIRONMENT AFTER BIRTH

Normal term neonates in bassinets should be dressed and blanketed. Table 10–2 shows the room air temperature necessary to provide adequate warmth for neonates kept clothed and well covered in a bassinet in a draught-free room of moderate (35%–60%) humidity.

Incubators

The air temperature of an incubator may be adjusted manually to provide an air temperature within the thermoneutral zone (Table 10–3). The manufacturer's recommended incubator air temperatures were determined in the laboratory under optimal conditions and should be used only as a general guide. The incubator air temperature should be recorded simultaneously with the neonate's axillary or skin temperature so that changes in the neonate's temperature can be interpreted appropriately. Plexiglas hemicylinders, bubble blankets, or double-walled incubators may be used to reduce heat loss from naked neonates inside incubators and are particularly useful for neonates weighing 1500 g or less.

Servocontrolled incubators generally need not be used in routine care so long as room temperature is reasonably stable, but neonates in incubators who are receiving phototherapy should have their skin temperature maintained at 36.5° C by means of a servocontrolled incubator. When servocontrol is used, the skin probe must be dry, taped securely to the exposed surface of the neonate, and protected from the light by an aluminum patch. Servocontrolled incubators can cause overheating if the skin sensor becomes loose.

High ambient humidity tends to encourage the growth of gram-negative bacilli on the skin, including *Escherichia coli* and *Pseudomonas*. On the other hand, high humidity tends to reduce insensible water

Table 10-2. *Room Temperature Required To Provide Adequate Warmth for Neonates*

Birth weight (kg)	Room temperature		
	29.5° C (85° F)	26.5° C (80° F)	24° C (75° F)
1.0	For 2 weeks	After 2 weeks	After 1 month
1.5	For 2 days	After 2 days	After 2 weeks
2.0		For 1 week	After 1 week
3.0		For 1 day	After 1 day

Table 10-3. Neutral Thermal Environmental Temperatures*

Age and weight	Starting temperature (°C)	Range of temperature (°C)
0–6 Hours		
Under 1200 g	35.0	34.0–35.4
1200–1500 g	34.1	33.9–34.4
1501–2500 g	33.4	32.8–33.8
Over 2500 (and > 36 weeks)	23.9	32.0–33.8
6–12 Hours		
Under 1200 g	35.0	34.0–35.4
1200–1500 g	34.0	33.5–34.4
1501–2500 g	33.1	32.2–33.8
Over 2500 (and > 36 weeks)	32.8	31.4–33.8
12–24 Hours		
Under 1200 g	34.0	34.0–35.4
1200–1500 g	33.8	33.3–34.3
1501–2500 g	32.8	31.8–33.8
Over 2500 (and > 36 weeks)	32.4	31.0–33.7
24–36 Hours		
Under 1200 g	34.0	34.0–35.0
1200–1500 g	33.6	33.1–34.2
1501–2500 g	32.6	31.6–33.6
Over 2500 (and > 36 weeks)	32.1	30.7–33.5
36–48 Hours		
Under 1200 g	34.0	34.0–35.0
1200–1500 g	33.5	33.0–34.1
1501–2500 g	32.5	31.4–33.5
Over 2500 (and > 36 weeks)	31.9	30.5–33.3
48–72 Hours		
Under 1200 g	34.0	34.0–35.0
1200–1500 g	33.5	33.0–34.0
1500–2500 g	32.3	31.2–33.4
Over 2500 (and > 36 weeks)	31.7	30.1–33.2
72–96 Hours		
Under 1200 g	34.0	34.0–35.0
1200–1500 g	33.5	33.0–34.0
1501–2500 g	32.2	31.1–33.2
Over 2500 (and > 36 weeks)	31.3	29.8–32.8
4–12 Days		
Under 1500 g	33.5	33.0–34.0
1501–2500 g	32.1	31.0–33.2
Over 2500 (and > 36 weeks)		
4–5 days	31.0	39.5–32.6
5–6 days	30.9	29.4–32.3
6–8 days	30.6	29.0–32.2
8–10 days	30.3	29.0–31.8
10–12 days	30.1	29.0–31.4
12–14 Days		
Under 1500 g	33.5	32.6–34.0
1501–2500 g	32.1	31.0–33.2
Over 2500 (and > 36 weeks)		
2–3 Weeks		
Under 1500 g	33.1	32.2–34.0
1501–2500 g	31.7	30.5–33.0

Table 10-3. *Neutral Thermal Environmental Temperatures* (continued)*

Age and weight	Starting temperature (°C)	Range of temperature (°C)
3–4 Weeks		
Under 1500 g	32.6	31.6–33.6
1501–2500 g	31.4	30.0–32.7
4–5 Weeks		
Under 1500 g	32.0	31.2–33.0
1501–2500 g	30.9	29.5–32.2
5–6 Weeks		
Under 1500 g	31.4	30.6–32.3
1501–2500 g	30.4	29.0–31.8

*Data from Scopes JW, Ahmed I: Minimal rates of oxygen consumption in sick and premature infants. Arch Dis Child 41:407–416, 1966; Scopes JW, Ahmed I: Range of critical temperatures in sick and premature newborn babies. Arch Dis Child:417–419, 1966. For his table, Scopes had the walls of the incubator 1° to 2° warmer than the ambient air temperatures.

Generally speaking, the smaller infants in each weight group require a temperature in the higher portion of the temperature range. Within each time range, the younger the infant, the higher the temperature required.

loss and evaporative heat loss. Available evidence suggests that a moderate relative humidity of about 50% provides optimal conditions for the neonate.

Radiant Warmers

Radiant warmers are frequently used because they facilitate contact with the neonate, particularly a critically ill neonate who requires cardiorespiratory support and monitoring or intensive care after surgery and various procedures. Neonates under radiant warmers have a significant increase in insensible water loss and a small increase in metabolic rate. These changes vary according to a neonate's weight and gestation, and no increase in fluid intake can be predetermined. Fluid requirements should be regulated according to clinical and biochemical criteria. Infection has not been found to be a significant problem for neonates nursed under these conditions.

Unless they are to be used for only a few minutes, these warmers should be used in the servocontrol mode with the abdominal skin temperature maintained at 36.5° C. The thermistor must be covered with an aluminum patch to prevent the radiant heat source from directly heating the thermistor, which should be securely taped to the anterior abdominal wall. Other potential dangers associated with the use of open radiant heaters include burns, unstable temperature control, difficulties using other equipment (e.g., x-ray, phototherapy), and overheating of staff working with the neonate.

HYPERTHERMIA

Infection, dehydration, and excessively high environmental temperature in improperly regulated incubators and radiant warmers, sometimes the result of improper placement of servocontrol probes, can all produce hyperthermia. Radiant heat from phototherapy lights and sunlight can overheat the neonate without (initially) warming the air in the surrounding environment. Measurement of the skin temperature of the anterior mid-lower leg simultaneously with the core temperature helps to differentiate pyrexia due to disease from that caused by environmental overheating. Hyperthermia increases metabolic demands and thus increases oxygen requirements and causes sweating in the full-term and older premature neonate.

Hyperthermia is treated by cooling the neonate as rapidly as possible. When the skin temperature is 37.5°–39° C, undressing and exposing the neonate to room temperature is usually all that is necessary. If the skin temperature is above 39° C, the patient should be undressed and sponged with tepid water at approximately 35° C until skin temperature is less than 38° C.

HYPOTHERMIA

Hypothermia is an abnormally low temperature, i.e., less than 36° C skin temperature and less than 36.5° C deep rectal or axillary temperature. Severe hypothermia compromises neonates. Hypothermic neonates appear red and edematous and may have sclerema. Lethargy, hypoglycemia, acidosis, azotemia, and pulmonary hemorrhage may also occur. Chronic, but mild, cold stress in the newborn increases metabolic rate and oxygen requirement, decreases growth rate, and may even be fatal.

The rate at which hypothermic neonates should be warmed is controversial. Fast warming has been shown to increase oxygen consumption, possibly causing apnea. Therefore, neonates should be monitored for metabolic acidosis, hypoglycemia, shock, clotting disorders, and hypoxia during warming. Blood pressure, blood glucose, pH and PaO_2 should also be monitored closely.

TEMPERATURE CONTROL IN SPECIAL CIRCUMSTANCES

Neonates with cyanotic cogenital heart disease may manifest aberrations in temperature control and are frequently diaphoretic, especially if they experience congestive heart failure. These neonates have a high metabolic rate and can easily become hyperthermic. Neonates born to mothers who have been given large doses of diazepam (Valium) have a blunted response to thermal stress, and hypothermia is common in these neonates. Thermolability, i.e., swings in body temperature, is more frequent then sustained temperature elevation in neonates with sepsis.

Inspired gas should be humidified and warmed to a temperature of 32°–36° C. The temperature of gas delivered to the neonate should be similar to that of the incubator temperature. Gases delivered directly via endotracheal tubes should be warmed to 35°–36° C.

In-house transport to and from facilities such as the operating room or radiology department may be done with a transport incubator or a regular incubator with the neonate lying on a heated mattress and covered by a thermal blanket. If a transport incubator is used, the air temperature should be set to approximate a thermoneutral environment. In cold environments, it is helpful to use a double-walled incubator in addition to covering the neonate with a thermal blanket. Transport incubators with radiant warming hoods are also effective. A similar system (or a circulating warm water mattress) can be used to keep the neonate's temperature stable during surgical procedures or computerized axial tomography (CAT) scans, radiologic procedures, and cardiac catheterization.

Since deaths and injuries due to hypothermia and hyperthermia have occurred, alarm systems and range controls of all equipment used for neonatal thermal regulators should be tested regularly. Nursery policies and procedures should specifically address this issue, and the time of testing should be documented.

Stillbirths, Neonatal Deaths, and Congenital Abnormalities

Families expect each child to be born healthy. Stillbirths, neonatal deaths, and congenital abnormalities are emotionally traumatic and require careful attention to management and counseling. A structured approach to these difficult clinical problems can help ease the guilt process and avoid prolonging the adjustment period confronted by parents in such cases.

STILLBIRTHS AND NEONATAL DEATHS

Late fetal death (stillbirth) occurs at 22 weeks or 500 g (see Definitions, Chapter 9). Approximately 1 in each 100 pregnancies greater than 20 weeks' gestation results in fetal demise. Etiology approximates one-half, fetal/placental structural or infective problems; one-fourth, congenital anomalies; and one-fourth, unknown. The emotional impact is greater than generally acknowledged in the recent past.

Each hospital should give careful thought to preparation of policies and procedures for dealing with stillbirth, including involvement of parents in seeing, touching, and holding their stillborn child. Many authorities feel that visual and physical contact within a professional environment may be very important to the process of reality testing, grief, and adjustment to future pregnancies. The obstetrician and pediatrician, individually or jointly, can and should play an important role in this process. In certain situations, the involvement of subspecialists such as geneticists or dysmorphologists may be important. In many areas, professional or lay support groups have been formed and can be very helpful.

Management

Proper management of stillbirth and neonatal death includes documentation of clinical findings, evaluation of the remains, appropriate laboratory studies, consultation with appropriate ancillary services, as well as proper counseling. A thorough diagnostic workup is important and justified for the parents' emotional well-being as well as for their guidance in regard to future pregnancies. A suggested protocol for this process is outlined in the following list:

1. Prenatal and family history. This evaluation should be complete, including detailed attention to family history.

2. Autopsy: fetus, placenta, and cord.

3. Photography. Total body photography is especially important if on-site dysmorphology consultation is not possible.

4. Total body x-rays. It is especially important to obtain x-rays of the skeletal structures if structural abnormalities or disproportion is suspected. In the future, whole body xerography may be helpful in some cases.

5. Cytogenetics. Heparinized blood from recent (less than 12 hours) stillbirths or neonatal deaths can be obtained from cord, peripheral vein, or the heart. Fibroblast cell cultures from dermis, tendon, or amnion may be obtained for up to 48 hours after death. Adherence to prior defined technique is important.

6. Bacterial and viral cultures and serologic studies.

7. Parent counseling.

Counseling

All parents who have had a stillborn or a newborn who has died in the neonatal period should be offered counseling, including genetic counseling when necessary. In addition, these parents require psychosocial support while they recover from the shock of the death.

Counseling should be both an immediate and an ongoing process, beginning at delivery, continuing through full discussion of test results when available, and if indicated, extending the next pregnancy. The following areas should be included:

Discussion of specific diagnosis or potential causes
Grief reaction
Guilt feelings
Consideration of future pregnancies

Frequently, parents demonstrate reactions of acute grief, such as somatic disturbances, a preoccupation with how the newborn looked or would have looked, guilt, hostility, and loss of ability to function. Mourning should be allowed to proceed. The staff should be aware that the parents are sensitive to the staff's reactions—frequently guilt, a sense of failure, and uncertainty—which may cause them to avoid the parents, thereby impeding discussion of the deceased infant with the family.

One member or a team of the staff—including either a physician, nurse, social worker, or members of the clergy—should be responsible for helping the parents:

1. Make the death a reality. Parents should be told that they may see and hold the dead newborn if they desire. The family should be helped in making funeral arrangements in accordance with their religious beliefs.

2. Work through the normal grief reaction. This is best accomplished by open discussion of the hopes, fears, and disappointments of the parents. Parents should be aware that their reaction of grief and hostility is normal; the hospital staff should understand the parents' feelings so they do not react in turn with hostility.

Follow-up sessions with the parents are often needed for continuing support and are recommended 2–6 weeks after the death. Parents without an extended family may gain strength from a parent support group at the hospital or in the community.

Legal Considerations

The death of a child in the perinatal period has legal, social, and emotional aspects that are confusing as well as sad. Perinatal staff should exercise extraordinary patience as they console and guide patients while explaining and complying with legal requirements. Staff members should be advised, however, not to respond definitively to patients' questions without first consulting the attending physician. Proper counseling can accomplish a great deal, including elimination of almost all points of confusion.

The following outline offers general guidance in this difficult area. Details will vary from state to state. The policies and procedures of each perinatal service should be reviewed.

For the live-born neonate who then expires (see Definitions, Chapter 9), the legal situation is identical to that of a deceased older child or adult:

1. Birth and death certificates must be completed.

2. In most states, the assistance of a funeral director whom the parents (or others taking responsibility for the body) choose is required for transportation of the body and arrangements for burial or cremation. The hospital may or may not be able to assume responsibility for final disposition of a live birth.

After a stillbirth, the parents in many locales have a choice of two legal modes for disposition of the body:

1. Burial or cremation by a funeral director as for a live birth.

2. Internal disposition by the hospital. If state laws permit, the remains

of a stillbirth are usually treated like human tissue removed at surgery; they are burned at a designated time in a designated place. This burning should not be described to the parents as "cremation" because, as all human tissue is burned together, parents cannot receive from the hospital the ashes of their child. (If the ashes were returned, this would constitute cremation and require a cremation permit issued only to funeral directors.) The cost of internal disposition may be borne by the hospital without funeral director expense.

In the usual cases of live birth or if the parents wish to receive the remains of a stillborn child, the family will probably require the services of a licensed funeral director. In most states, a body cannot be transported except by a funeral director or perhaps by relatives who have complied with a delineated policy. Burial in a place other than a cemetery is possible but complicated. (The funeral director can be helpful in arranging this.)

A funeral director need not be chosen for a few hours. Funeral directors usually accept calls asking for advice or referral and will arrange to talk to the family in person or by telephone at a reasonable hour even after the parents have returned to their home.

Parents' questions regarding cost of burial, cremation, and transport of remains should be referred to a funeral director unless the physician or nurse is knowledgeable about details and recent laws and regulations. Licensed funeral directors are trained to counsel families regarding their options and costs; costs change rather dramatically from time to time, and an outdated answer from a hospital staff member can have disappointing consequences. The social worker assigned to the perinatal service may be an excellent resource when working with families in these difficult circumstances.

CONGENITAL ABNORMALITIES

After 20 weeks of gestation, 1.6% of all fetuses have a serious multi-factorial, chromosomal, or mendelian malformation. Approximately 22% of these die soon after birth. Since the phenotypic expression of these malformations is frequently nonconclusive, laboratory or autopsy findings are essential to understanding the disease.

It is important that the parents of a neonate with congenital malformations or genetic abnormalities have a clear understanding of the precise problems, need (or lack of need) for therapy, future prognosis, and appropriate future therapeutic modalities. Parental guilt because of real or imagined exposure or influences during the pregnancy should be allayed, if possible. Care for both the neonate and family should be individualized, and social workers should participate in the supportive effort.

The parents should receive appropriate genetic counseling on the hereditary factors associated with the congenital abnormality and the risk of recurrence in a subsequent pregnancy. This counseling attempts to help the family (1) comprehend the medical facts, (2) appreciate the inheritance pattern and risks of recurrence, (3) understand the options for dealing with recurrence, (4) choose a course of action, and (5) adjust to the disorder. Counseling requires a sensitive approach on the part of the physician if the family is to understand and accept the discussion. When some aspect of genetic counseling is beyond the expertise of the neonatologist or pediatrician, consultation with a geneticist is essential.

Adoption

Complex medical, legal, and social problems might be encountered in an adoption, and physicians involved in placing the adoptive newborn should be familiar with the proper procedures.

ADOPTION PROCEDURES

Most adopted newborns originate from out-of-wedlock pregnancies. An estimated 665,747 babies were born out of wedlock in 1980, compared with 399,000 in 1970, according to the National Center for Health Statistics. The 1980 figure represents 18.4% of all births, compared with 10.7% in 1970. Although more babies are being born out of wedlock, the majority of single mothers choose to keep their babies, and the number of couples who wish to adopt is increasing. Even though the demand for babies far exceeds the supply, it is possible for a determined couple to adopt a baby or a very young child.

Couples often first turn to the obstetrician-gynecologist for advice concerning adoption. In addition, adoption agencies look to obstetricians to give conscientious and thorough appraisal of the applicants' physical and emotional capacity for becoming parents. If the couple is seeking an adoption because of primary or secondary infertility, it is assumed that both parents have had a complete workup and that the alternatives, such as donor or husband insemination, have been discussed with them. The physician should understand that the couple may need help in overcoming the grief and anger that frequently result from the inability to conceive a child.

Once a couple has reached the decision to seek a child via adoption, they are usually anxious and impatient to get the procedure under way. The physician should explain realistically what is involved in an adoption and the time required. Both social welfare and private agencies are good resources, and the physician should make referrals. The couple should be informed that the agencies must follow certain procedures, including an investigation of the couple who wish to adopt. The couple should be encouraged to reexamine their own motives for adoption and also to familiarize themselves with the legal steps necessary for valid adoption.

Easing patients through the maze of decisions and regulations that they will face if they choose to adopt is not a clinician's traditional role. Adoption is a legal, not a medical, process; hence, the physician is not the best person to handle an adoption directly. However, the physician is the most suitable individual to advise and refer the couple to the best resources available. It is essential that physicians, nurses, and medical social workers involved in the adoption have a thorough knowledge of local procedures, resources, and the legal process of the laws and regulations regarding adoption in their state.

Each state has its own body of laws, rules, and regulations covering adoption. Every state requires an assessment of adoptive parents, and most states have specific residency requirements. In most other respects, however, there is a notable lack of uniformity. For example, some states permit direct contact with birth parents, while other states do not. Since adoption laws vary greatly from state to state, adoptive parents are wise to choose an agency within their own state, avoiding the complications associated with interstate placement laws.

To an agency, the safeguards for the child, the birth parents, and the adoptive parents are foremost. Agencies not only offer preparation for adoptive parenthood but also provide counseling and support services to the birth mother to protect her from making an unwise or hasty decision. Likewise, through careful home study, agencies reduce the danger of a child being inappropriately placed. In addition, agencies ensure that physicians and adoptive parents do not inadvertently break the law.

Independent adoptions are legal in some states. In such cases, prospective adoptive parents may pay for the pregnant woman's food, housing, and medical care; any additional payment is strictly prohibited, however. In many states, intervention by a third party is also illegal, and a physician or lawyer who acts as an intermediary is liable for prosecution.

Every adoption should be handled by a lawyer; two lawyers are often required when the adoptive family and the child are in different states. Experienced lawyers and adoption agencies protect the rights of both the birth and adoptive parents and ensure that the adoption is properly executed, thus avoiding subsequent charge.

After the birth of the adoptive baby, certain procedures should be followed to serve the best interest of the birth mother, the newborn, and the adoptive parents, as well as to promote continuity of care.

Nursery Observation

Adoptive newborns should be united as soon as possible with the new parents. A period of at least 48, and preferably 72, hours of in-hospital observation is desirable to ensure that the neonate is stabilized fully. Guidelines cited in Chapter 4 should be followed. Some state laws do not allow the adoptive newborn to be placed with the adoptive parents until 48 hours after birth, and usually agencies will not place newborns less than 3 days old.

Nursing and medical observations of the adoptive newborn should be identical to those received by any newborn. The laboratory evaluation of the neonate should be determined by basic medical needs, not by the adoption process. Results of all tests not available at discharge should be reported to the agency and the physician who will have continuing medical responsibility for the newborn.

Physicians and nurses should be sensitive to the birth mother's needs and desires. She should be encouraged to see her newborn at least once. If she desires, the birth mother should be informed of any problems related to the baby. The birth mother should be reminded that she has the right to have this contact with her newborn, although she should not be overly pressured to do so.

Physical Evaluation of Adoptive Neonate

The physician's responsibility is to assess the newborn's present status, perform appropriate risk assessment to identify problems that may arise later in life, and report this information to the agency or family for their careful consideration. When medical problems have been identified and adoption is to proceed, disclosure should be complete, including estimates of possible treatment, prognosis, and extent of care. Complete medical documentation should be provided to the placement resource. Questions concerning the condition and care of the neonate should be answered fully.

Following a thorough review of the obstetric chart and the family history, a check of the birth mother's wishes, and a conference with the social worker, the physician should convey a brief review of the newborn's status to the birth mother. If additional data (e.g., the potential for substance withdrawal) or clarification of a physical finding or behavior of the newborn is needed, further discussion with the birth mother may be necessary.

RESPONSIBILITY TO THE BIRTH MOTHER

Use of an adoption communication sheet (see example in Appendix I) facilitates consistent, sensitive care during the perinatal period.

1. Care should be maintained not to disclose the birth mother's identity to the adoptive parents if the baby is to be placed through an agency.

2. An obstetric social worker should assess the birth mother's feelings concerning adoption plans.
3. It should be remembered that, whatever the birth mother's original intent, some ambivalence may be normal and she may see and hold her baby until she has formally waived parental rights.
4. Nursing and medical care of the birth mother should be identical to that received by other new mothers.

RESPONSIBILITY TO THE ADOPTIVE PARENTS

Adoptive parents have no right to contact their new baby without appropriate legal clearance. When legal clearance has been obtained, hospital personnel should facilitate contact between adoptive parents and their baby. In some states, however, legal clearance is not given until at least 30 days after birth; the child is placed in a foster home in the interim.

If the law allows the adopting parents to visit the neonate in the hospital, the wishes of birth parents should not be overshadowed by the wishes of the adoptive parents. In states where direct placement is possible, visits by the adoptive parents in the hospital should be considered. Parents adopting through direct placement may know the identity of the birth parents in some situations. In states where this is not allowed, care should be taken to preserve anonymity.

The need of the adoptive parents to learn parenting skills should be recognized and honored. Prospective parents should be encouraged to attend child care classes.

RESOURCES AND RECOMMENDED READING

Antenatal Detection of Genetic Disorders

Alter B: Prenatal diagnosis of haemoglobinopathies: A status report. Lancet 2:(8256)1152–1154, 1981

American Academy of Pediatrics Committee on Genetics: Prenatal diagnosis for pediatricians. Pediatrics 65(6):1185–1186, 1980

American College of Obstetricians and Gynecologists: Antenatal Diagnosis of Genetic Disorders (Technical Bulletin 39). Washington, DC, ACOG, 1976

An Assessment of the Hazards of Amniocentesis. Report to the Medical Research Council by Their Working Party on Amniocentesis. Br J Obstet Gynecol 85 (2 suppl):2:1–41, 1978

Burton BK, Nadler HL: Antenatal diagnosis of metabolic disorders. Clin Obstet Gynecol 24(4):1041–1054, 1981

Chang JC, Kan YW: Antenatal diagnosis of sickle cell anemia by direct analysis of the sickle mutation. Lancet 2(8256):1127–1129, 1981

Hamerton JL, Simpson NE (eds): Prenatal diagnosis: Past, present and future. Prenatal Diagnosis 1 (special issue): 1–63, 1980

Hobbins J, Grannum P, Berkowitz RL, et al: Ultrasound in the diagnosis of congenital anomalies. Am J Obstet Gynecol 134(3):331–345, 1979

Milunsky A (ed): Genetic Disorders and the Fetus. New York, Plenum Press, 1979

Murken JA, Stengel-Rugkowski S, Schwinger E: Prenatal Diagnosis. Proceedings of the 3rd European Conference on Prenatal Diagnosis of Genetic Disorders. Littleton, MA, John Wright, Inc, 1978

Nadler HL (ed): Antenatal assessment of genetic defects, growth retardation and fetal maturity. Semin Perinatol 4(3):157–247, 1980

NICHD National Registry for Amniocentesis Study Group: Midtrimester amniocentesis for prenatal diagnosis: Safety and accuracy. JAMA 236(13):1471–1476, 1976

Simpson JL: Antenatal diagnosis of cytogenetic abnormalities. Clin Obstet Gynecol 24(4):1023–1054, 1981

Simpson JL (ed): Antenatal detection of genetic disorders. Clin Obstet Gynecol 24:1005–1171, 1981

Simpson JL, Elias S, Gatlin MJ, et al: Genetic counseling and genetic services in obstetrics and gynecology: Implications for educational goals and clinical practice. Am J Obstet Gynecol 140(1):70–80, 1981

Simpson NE, Dallaire L, Miller JR, et al: Prenatal diagnosis of genetic disease in Canada: Report of a collaborative study. Can Med Assoc J 115(8):739–748, 1976

US Department of Health, Education, and Welfare; Public Health Service, National Institutes of Health: Antenatal Diagnosis NIH Publication No. 79-1973. Washington DC, US Government Printing Office, 1979

Hyperbilirubinemia

Brodersen R: Binding of bilirubin to albumin. CRC Crit Rev Clin Lab Sci 11(4):305–399, 1980

Cashore WJ, Oh W: Unbound bilirubin and kernicterus in low-birthweight infants. Pediatrics 69(4):481–485, 1982

Crichton JU, Dunn HG, McBurney AK, et al: Long-term effects of neonatal jaundice on brain function in children of very low birth weight. Pediatrics 49:656–670, 1972

Diamond I, Schmid R: Experimental bilirubin encephalopathy: The mode of entry of bilirubin-^{14}C into the central nervous system. J Clin Invest 45:678–689, 1966

Hammerman C, Eidelman AI, Lee K-S, et al: Comparative measurements of phototherapy: A practical guide. Pediatrics 67(3):368–372, 1981

Hsia DY-Y, Allen IH, Gellis SS, et al: Erythroblastosis fetalis: VIII. Studies of serum bilirubin in relation to kernicterus. N Engl J Med 247(18):668–671, 1952

Johnson L, Boggs TR: Bilirubin-dependent brain damage: Incidence and indications for treatment. In: Odell GB, Schaffer R, Simopoulous AP (eds): Phototherapy in the Newborn: An overview. Washington, DC, National Academy of Sciences, 1974, pp 122–149

Kim MH, Yoon JJ, Sher J, et al: Lack of predictive indices in kernicterus: A comparison of clinical and pathologic factors in infants with or without kernicterus. Pediatrics 66(6):852–858, 1980

Levine RL, Fredericks WR, Rapoport SI: Entry of bilirubin into the brain due to opening of the blood-brain barrier. Pediatrics 69(3):255–259, 1982

Naeye RL: Amniotic fluid infections, neonatal hyperbilirubinemia and psychomotor impairment. Pediatrics 62(4):497–503, 1978

Ritter DA, Kenny JD, Norton HJ, et al: A prospective study of free bilirubin and other risk factors in the development of kernicterus in premature infants. Pediatrics 69(3):260–266, 1982

Rubin RA, Balow B, Fisch RO: Neonatal serum bilirubin levels related to cognitive development at ages 4 through 7 years. J Pediatr 94(4):601–604, 1979

Shiller JG, Silverman WA: "Uncomplicated" hyperbilirubinemia of prematurity: The lack of association with neurologic deficit at 3 years of age. Am J Dis Child 101:587–592, 1961

Tan KL: Comparison of the effectiveness of phototherapy and exchange transfusion in the management of nonhemolytic neonatal hyperbilirubinemia. J Pediatr 87(4):609–612,1975

Tan KL: The nature of the dose-response relationship of phototherapy for neonatal hyperbilirubinemia. J Pediatr 90(3):448–452, 1977

Turkel SB, Guttenberg ME, Moynes DR, et al: Lack of identifiable risk factors for kernicterus. Pediatrics 66(4):502–506, 1980

Turkel SB, Miller CA, Guttenberg ME, et al: A clinical pathologic reappraisal of kernicterus. Pediatrics 69(3):267–272, 1982

Wennberg RP, Depp R, Heinrichs WL: Indications for early exchange transfusion in patients with erythroblastosis fetalis. J Pediatr 92(5):789–792, 1978

Wishingrad L, Cornblath M, Takakuwa P, et al: Studies of non-hemolytic hyperbilirubinemia in premature infants. I. Prospective randomized selection for exchange transfusion with observations on the levels of serum bilirubin with and without exchange transfusion and neurologic evaluations one year after birth. Pediatrics 36:162–172, 1965

Thermal Regulation

Day RL, Caliguiri L, Kamenski C, et al: Body temperature and survival of premature infants. Pediatrics 34:171–181, 1964

Fleischman AR: Another potential hazard of radiant warmers. J Pediatr 91(6):984, 1977

Hey EN: Thermal regulation in the newborn. Br J Hosp Med 8:51–64, 1972

Kennaird DL: Oxygen consumption and evaporative water loss in infants with congenital heart disease. Arch Dis Child 51(1)34–41, 1976

Marks KH, Friedman Z, Maisels MJ: A simple device for reducing insensible water loss in low-birth-weight infants. Pediatrics 60(2):223–226, 1977

Marks KH, Gunther RC, Rossi JA, et al: Oxygen consumption and insensible water loss in premature infants under radiant heaters. Pediatrics 66(2):228–232, 1980

Marks KH, Lee CA, Bolan CD Jr, et al: Oxygen consumption and temperature control of premature infants in a double-wall incubator. Pediatrics 68(1):93–98, 1981

McLaughlin JF, Telzrow RW, Scott CM: Neonatal mercury vapor exposure in an infant incubator. Pediatrics 66(6):988–990, 1980

Pleet H, Graham JM Jr, Smith DW: Central nervous system and facial defects associated with maternal hyperthermia at four to 14 weeks' gestation. Pediatrics 67(6):785–789, 1981

Pomerance JJ, Brand RJ, Meredith JL: Differentiating environmental from disease-related fevers in the term newborn. Pediatrics 67(4):485–488, 1981

Rutter N, Brown SM, Hull D: Variations in the resting oxygen consumption of small babies. Arch Dis Child. 53(11):850–854, 1978

Silverman WA, Sinclair JC: Temperature regulation in the newborn infant. N Engl J Med. 274:92–94, 146–148, 1966

Sinclair JC: Metabolic rate and temperature control. In Smith CA, Nelson NM (eds): The physiology of the newborn infant. Springfield, IL, Charles C Thomas, 1976, pp 4, ed 354–415

Smales OR, Kime R: Thermoregulation in babies immediately after birth. Arch Dis Child. 53(1):58–61, 1978

Waffarn F, Hodgman JE: Mercury vapor contamination of infant incubators: A potential hazard. Pediatrics 64(5):640–642, 1979

Adoption

American Academy of Pediatrics, Committee on Adoption and Dependent Care: The role of the pediatrician in adoption with reference to "the right to know": An update. Pediatrics 67(2):305–306, 1981

American Academy of Pediatrics, Committee on Adoption and Dependent Care: Intercountry adoption. Pediatrics 68(4):596–597, 1981

American Academy of Pediatrics, Committee on Adoption and Dependent Care: Adoption of the hard-to-place child. Pediatrics 68(4):598–599, 1981

Baran A, Pannor R, Sorosky A: The lingering pain of surrendering a child. Psychology Today 11(1):58, 1977

Concerned United Birthparents: Understanding the Birthparent. Milford, MA, CUB, 1977

Fisch RO, Bilek MK, Deinara AS, et al: Growth, behavioral and psychologic measurements of adopted children: The influences of genetic and socioeconomic factors in a prospective study. J Pediatr 89(3):494–500, 1976

Frank DA, Graham JM, Smith DW: (Letter) Adoptive children in a dysmorphology clinic: Implications for evaluation of children before adoption. Pediatrics 68(5):744–745, 1981

Quinn NJ Jr, et al: Operation Stork: Promoting infant-maternal bonding with adopting parents. Clin Pediatr 17(8):652–658, 1978

Smith J: You're Our Child. Wolfe City, TX University Press, 1981

Sokoloff B: Adoption and foster care—The pediatrician's role. Pediatrics 64(2):PIR 57–61, 1979

Appendix

A
Illustrative Categorization of Perinatal Services

The following matrix is offered to assist individual regional programs in the process of organization. The broad goals identified in Chapter 1 (reduction of perinatal mortality and morbidity, efficient utilization of resources) should be linked to specific individualized service, education, research, and administrative objectives that are locally determined. The local effort can modify specific parts of the matrix according to needs and resources. The guidelines given here and, in greater detail, in Chapters 2 (Physical Facilities) and 3 (Personnel) are probably reasonable and attainable in most regions.

Table A-1. Perinatal Care Programs

	Level I	Level II	Level III
Function	Risk assessment Management of uncomplicated perinatal care Stabilization of unexpected problems Initiation of maternal and neonatal transports Patient and community education Data collection and evaluation	*General* Level I plus: Diagnosis and treatment of selected high-risk pregnancies and neonatal problems Initiation and acceptance of maternal-fetal and neonatal transports Education of allied health personnel Residency education (affiliation)	Levels I and II plus: Diagnosis and treatment of all perinatal problems Acceptance and direction of maternal-fetal and neonatal transports Research and outcome surveillance Graduate and postgraduate education System management
Types of patients	Uncomplicated, emergency, and remedial problems such as lack of progress, immediate resuscitation of asphyxiated neonates, uterine atony, nursery care of large premature neonates (> 2000 g) without risk factors, physiologic jaundice	Level I plus: Selected problems such as preeclampsia, premature labor at 32 weeks and later, mild to moderate respiratory distress syndrome, suspected neonatal sepsis, hypoglycemia, neonates of diabetic mothers, postasphyxia without life-threatening sequalae	Levels I and II plus: Premature rupture of membranes at 24–26 weeks, severe maternal medical complications, pregnancy with concurrent cancer, complicated antenatal genetic problems, prematurity at 26–32 weeks (500–1250 g), severe respiratory distress syndrome, sepsis, severe postasphyxia, symptomatic congenital cardiac and other systems disease, neonates with special needs such as hyperalimentation, prolonged mechanical ventilation

continued

Table A-1. *Perinatal Care Programs (continued)*

	Level I	Level II	Level III
Location and number of births, neonatal beds	Located within Level II or III hospital or in sparsely populated or isolated areas; at least 1 birth/day unless in isolated area	Medium and large communities, may be part of Level III facility, several births/day, 3–4 neonatal beds/1000 births served	Medium and large communities, usually in academic centers, several births/day, 1 intensive care neonatal bed/1000 births served in addition to Level II
Sq ft/bed	Delivery/resuscitation 120 Admission/observation 40 Newborn nursery 20 Postpartum unit 100	*Space* Level I plus: Intermediate nursery 50 Continuous/convalescent nursery 30	Levels I and II plus: Intensive neonatal 80–100
Chief of Service	One physician responsible for perinatal care (or co-directors from obstetrics and pediatrics)	*Personnel* Joint planning: *Ob*: Board-certified obstetrician with certification, special interest, experience, or training in maternal-fetal medicine; *Peds*: Board-certified pediatrician with certification, special interest, experience or training in neonatology	Codirectors: *Ob*: Full-time board-certified obstetrician with special competence in maternal-fetal medicine; *Peds*: Full-time board-certified pediatrician with special competence in neonatal medicine
Other physicians	Physician (or certified nurse-midwife) at all deliveries, Anesthesia services Physician care for neonates	Level I plus: Board-certified director of anesthesia services Medical, surgical, radiology, pathology consultation	Levels I and II plus: Anesthesiologists with special training or experience in perinatal and pediatric anesthesia Obstetric and pediatric subspecialists

	Level I	Level II	Level III
		experience in normal and high-risk pregnancy only responsible	with advanced skills
		Peds: RN with education and experience in treatment of sick neonates only responsible	Separate head nurses for maternal-fetal and neonatal services
Staff nurse/patient ratio	Normal labor 1:2 Delivery in second stage 1:1 Oxytocin inductions 1:2 Cesarean delivery 2:1 Normal nursery 1:6–8	Level I plus: Complicated labor/delivery 1:1 Intermediate nursery 1:3–4	Levels I and II plus: Intensive neonatal care 1:1–2 Critical care of unstable neonate 2:1
Other personnel	LPN, assistants under direction of head nurse	Level I plus: Social service, biomedical, respiratory therapy, laboratory as needed	Levels I plus: Designated and often full-time social service, respiratory therapy, biomedical engineering, laboratory technician Nurse-clinician and specialists Nurse program and education coordinators

Obstetric Units

	Level I	Level II	Level III
Admission/observation	Close to labor and delivery, comfortable, room to ambulate	Level I plus: Beds, space for diagnostic procedures, possible emergency delivery	Levels I and II plus: Other bed designated for observation
Family waiting	Nearby/adjacent	Level I	Level I
Labor	Single: 140 sq ft multiple, 80 sq ft/ patient Beds adjustable and moveable to delivery, may be used as birthing bed Full utilities, including auxiliary electrical, oxygen, suction Communication system Full routine patient care and CPR equipment Secure medication area Monitoring capabilities	Level I	Level I

continued

	Level I	Level II	Level III
Birthing (labor/delivery/recovery)	Combined equipment for labor and delivery, may be concealed Adequate space, equipment for ambulation, support person	Level I	Level I
Delivery (vaginal and operative)	Contiguous to labor; at least two available, with one equipped for cesarean delivery Operating room in design Equipment/supplies necessary for normal delivery and management of complications, including surgical intervention	Level I (Actual number of delivery rooms depends on total births) plus: Intensive care room in labor/delivery area for patients with significant complication	Levels I and II plus: Intensive care area
Antepartum and postpartum area	Contiguous with nursery Large enough to accommodate mother, baby, visitors Maximum two mothers/room 100 sq ft/patient in multiple patient rooms Communication system Hospital standard utilities	Level I	Level I
Resuscitation	100 foot-candles illumination Overhead radiant heat Heating pad Wall clock Resuscitation and stabilization equipment Designated area (40 sq ft) or room (120 sq ft) Full utilities, including suction, oxygen, compressed air, electrical outlets	*Nursery* Level I	Level I

Admission/observation	Near or adjacent to delivery/cesarean birth room, may be part of maternal recovery area 40 sq ft/neonate Equipment as in resuscitation area	May be located in newborn or continuing care area	Level II
Newborn nursery	Close to postpartum area Beds and equipment to exceed obstetric beds by 20%–30% 20 sq ft/neonate Resuscitation equipment 1 electrical outlet/2 beds 1 O_2, air suction/5–6 beds	Level I	Level I
Continuing care	Usually not located in Level I	Near intermediate nursery. 30 sq ft/neonate Resuscitation equipment 4 electrical outlets 1 O_2, 1 air, 1 suction/neonate	Level II
Intermediate care	Not present	Near delivery and intensive care nurseries Full life support and monitoring in addition to resuscitation equipment 50 sq ft/neonate 8 electrical, 2 O_2, 2 compressed air, 2 suction outlets/neonate	Level II
Intensive care	Not present	Present in some hospitals	Near delivery/cesarean birth rooms 80–100 sq ft/neonate 12 electrical, 2 O_2, 2 compressed air, 2 suction outlets/neonate Full life support, monitoring and resuscitation equipment
Operating room	Technicians on call 24 h/day, available within 15–30 min	*Ancillary Support* Technicians immediately available for emergency situations	Level II, may be in delivery room area

continued

Table A-1. Perinatal Care Programs

	Level I	Level II	Level III
Laboratory (microtechnique for neonates)			
Within 15 min	Hematocrit	Blood gases, blood type and Rh	Level II
Within 1 h	Glucose, BUN, creatinine, blood gases, routine urinalysis	Level I plus: Electrolytes, coagulation studies, blood available from Type and Screen program	Levels I and II plus: Special blood and amniotic fluid tests
Within 1–6 hr	CBC, platelet appearance on smear, blood chemistries, blood type and cross matched, Coombs' test, bacterial smear	Level I plus: Coagulation studies, magnesium, urine, electrolytes, and chemistries	Levels I and II
Within 24–48 hr	Bacterial cultures and antibiotic sensitivity	Level I plus: Liver function test, Metabolic screening	Levels I and II
Within hospital or facilities available	Viral cultures	Level I	Level I plus: Laboratory facilities available
Radiography and ultrasound	Technicians on call 24 hr/day, available in 30 min Technicians experienced in performing abdominal, pelvic and OB ultrasound examinations Professional interpretation available on 24 hr basis Portable x-ray and ultrasound equipment available to labor and delivery rooms and to nurseries	Experienced radiology technicians immediately available in hospital (ultrasound on call) Professional interpretation immediately available Portable x-ray equipment Ultrasound equipment may be in labor and delivery or nursery areas Sophisticated equipment for emergency GI, GU or CNS studies available 24 hr/day	Level II plus: Computerized axial tomography

	Level I	Level II	Level III
Blood bank	Technicians on call 24 hr/day, available in 30 min, performing routine blood banking procedures	Experienced technicians immediately available in hospital for blood banking procedures and identification of irregular antibodies Blood component therapy readily available	Level II plus: Resource center for network Direct line communication to labor and delivery area and nurseries
Examination and treatment room	Pelvic examination Culture of cervix and uterus	Level I plus: Amniocentesis Equipment for removal of suture for cerclage	Levels I and II plus: Services within unit
Auxiliary areas	Parent education Conference room Locker room (may be remote) Physician on-call room nearby	Level I plus: Breast-feeding area within unit Parent waiting room for intensive care	Levels I and II plus: All areas within unit Conference/lecture rooms as necessary for professional/regional education commitments
	Laboratory within unit for hematocrit, centrifuge for dip stick for urine, albumin, glucose, microscope	Level I plus: Refrigerator to hold cultures, materials Gram stain material	Levels I and II

B

Equipment and Supplies for Resuscitation

A. General
1. EKG machine
2. Ice maker
3. Ultrasound blood pressure detector (one per six patients)
4. Refractometer
5. Hampers for clean and dirty laundry
6. Soap and towel dispensers
7. Wastebaskets with disposable linings
8. Chart racks
9. Neonate scales, 10 kg
10. 500-g scales
11. Wall clocks with sweep second hand
12. Refrigerators
13. Instrument stands
14. Supply carts
15. Surgical trays
    a. Umbilical vessel catheterization
    b. Thoracostomy
    c. Exchange transfusion
    d. Circumcision
16. Surgical instruments
    a. Scissors
    b. Adsin forceps
    c. Hemostats
    d. Knife handles
    e. McGill forceps
    f. Surgical blades
17. Compressed air and oxygen (warmed and humidified)
18. Ventilation bag, 500 ml flow-through with adjustable pop-off valve capable of generating pressure of 40–50 mm H_2

B. Individual Patient
1. Incubators
2. Incubator scales
3. Radiant heat
4. Heating mattresses
5. Heart rate/respirator/blood pressure monitors
6. Blood pressure transducers
7. Infusion pumps
8. Intravenous stands
9. Oxygen-air blenders
10. Gas flow meters (oxygen and air)
11. Oxygen analyzers
12. Oxygen humidifier/nebulizer with heater
13. Oxygen temperature detector and alarm
14. Oxygen hoods
15. Suction pressure regulators
16. Suction/drainage bottles
17. Wastebaskets
18. Charts (bedside and physicians'/nurses' stations)

C. Supplies
1. Surgical gloves/finger cots
2. Blood culture tubes
3. Alcohol swabs and solution
4. Providone iodine swabs and solution
5. Cotton balls
6. Thermometers and lubricant
7. Culture swabs and media
8. Sponges
9. Medicine cups
10. Safety pins
11. Sutures
12. Adhesive tape
13. Syringes and needles
14. Intravenous infusion sets and tubing
15. Wash basin for bathing the neonate
16. Infant soap and lotion
17. Charting forms (bedside and physicians'/nurses' stations)
18. Requisition forms
19. Liquid hand-washing soap
20. Surgical soap sponges
21. Fingernail cleaners
22. Paper towels

23. Labstix
24. Dextrostix
25. Disposable tape measures
26. Lancets
27. Microscope slides
28. Cotton-tipped applicators
29. Urine collection bags
30. Rubber bands
31. Diapers, both cloth and disposable
32. Surgical cover gowns
33. Bed linen
34. Suction catheters #6, 7, 10 and 12 Fr
35. Feeding tubes #5 and 8 Fr
36. Replogle tubes #12 Fr
37. Equipment for performing hematocrit
38. Ventilation bag, 500-ml self-inflating type with attachment to ensure delivery of 100% oxygen, or 500-ml anesthesia bag with appropriate elbow and pressure manometer
39. Face masks, neonate sizes 1–4 (Bird) or O and OA (Ambu)
40. Stethoscope
41. Neonate laryngoscope with pencil handle and 0 and 1 straight blades, spare batteries, and bulbs
42. Endotracheal tubes, sterile and disposable, sizes 2.5, 3, 3.5, 4 mm with malleable stylets (tubes designated IT [implantation tested] or Z79 meet with the required standards)

C
Preconceptional Care

Preparation for parenthood should begin prior to conception. At the time of conception the couple should be in optimal physical health and emotionally prepared for parenthood. In order to make an informed decision about parenthood, a couple should have a realistic assessment of their mental and physical status and a thorough explanation of the risks associated with a prospective pregnancy.

When pregnancy is contemplated, preconceptual counseling should be part of a comprehensive gynecologic examination. This examination should include a detailed family history of any unusual or abnormal births within the immediate or extended family. An extensive checklist, such as that shown in the following example, should be used to outline the family's background, lifestyle, religion, ethnic background, home and work environment, hobbies, pets, immunizations, medications, and dietary habits. From this information a general counseling and instruction session may focus on the following areas:

1. Testing for a carrier state or other predisposing factor (e.g., Tay-Sachs carrier screening in prospective parents, blood and Rh type in a woman prior to pregnancy, serology, and rubella antibody titer)

2. Problems that can and should be resolved prior to pregnancy (e.g., anemia)

3. Problems that cannot be resolved, but may require extra care prior to and during pregnancy

4. The recurrence of complications experienced in previous pregnancies, including congenital anomalies

5. The length of time to wait after use of oral contraceptives or spontaneous or induced abortion

6. Problems associated with potential teratogenic effects of prescribed medications, illicit substances, alcohol, and smoking

7. Exercise and diet in pregnancy

8. The importance of recording the data of each menstrual period and beginning prenatal care as early as possible in the course of pregnancy

Preconception Inventory

Patient name _____ Age _____ Wife _____ Husband _____
Patient address _____ Telephone _____
Referring physician _____
Referring physician address _____ Telephone _____
Religion _____ Ethnic background _____ Blood type _____
Receives regular health care by _____
Reason for seeking preconception counseling _____

Family history

_____ Diabetes (relationship to patient _____
_____ Hypertension (relationship to patient) _____
_____ Epilepsy (relationship to patient) _____
_____ Multiple pregnancies (relationship to patient) _____
_____ Other (specify) _____
_____

Genetic history

Has the patient been screened for special disease relating to ethnic background?
_____ yes _____ no If yes, explain _____
Is there any family history of: (Include previous children by either parent)
_____ Muscular dystrophy (relationship to patient) _____
_____ Hemophilia (relationship to patient) _____
_____ Cystic fibrosis (relationship to patient) _____
_____ Mental retardation (relationship to patient) _____
_____ Birth defects (relationship to patient) _____
_____ Short stature (relationship to patient) _____
Is there anything that the patient is especially concerned about? _____
_____
_____
_____

Medical history

_____ Diabetes: Onset? _____
_____ Hypertension: Onset? _____ Range? _____
_____ Epilepsy: Onset? _____
_____ Anemia: For how long? _____
_____ Rubella: When? _____
_____ Menses: Onset? _____ Regular _____
_____ Surgery: if so, what type? _____
_____ Contraception: Methods used? _____
_____ Accidents: What type? _____
_____ Allergies: What type? _____
_____ Immunizations: _____

Preconception Inventory (cont.)

Current medication

General: (including over-the-counter drugs) _____
_____

Specific:

_____ Oral contraceptives: Type _____ Duration _____
_____ Sedatives or Tranquilizers: _____
_____ Drugs: _____
_____ Alcohol: _____ Beer _____ Wine _____ Liquor _____
_____ Smoking: _____ Packs per day _____
_____ Snuff: _____
_____ Appetite suppressants _____
_____ Diuretics _____
_____ Antibiotics _____
_____ Caffeine: _____
_____ Drugs of abuse _____

Nutrition

Present status:

Height _____   Weight _____

Does the patient make an effort to control weight?   _____ yes _____ no
Does the patient take vitamins?   _____ yes _____ no
   If yes, which ones? _____
Is the patient a vegetarian?   _____ yes _____ no
   If yes, what type? _____

Environmental factors

Occupation _____
Hobbies _____
Source of water supply _____
Pets _____ Exercise _____

Obstetric history

Gravida _____ Para _____
Deliveries _____ Management _____
Surgery _____
Pregnancy complications _____

Counseling

Specialized _____

Comments

_____
_____

D

Sample List of Perinatal Conditions That Increase the Risk for Neonatal Morbidity or Mortality

SECTION A

Conditions Requiring Availability of Skilled Resuscitation at Delivery

1. Fetal distress
   a. Persistent late decelerations
   b. Severe variable decelerations without baseline variability
   c. Scalp pH $\leq$ 7.25
   d. Meconium-stained amniotic fluid
   e. Cord prolapse
2. Operative delivery
   a. Cesarean delivery
   b. Mid-forceps delivery
3. Third trimester bleeding
4. Multiple births
5. Estimated birth weight $\leq$ 1500 g
6. Estimated gestational age $\leq$ 34 weeks
7. Breech presentation
8. Prolonged, unusual, or difficult labor
9. Insulin-dependent diabetes
10. Severe isoimmunization
11. Obstetrician's or pediatrician's request

SECTION B

Conditions Requiring an Immediate Assessment and Initiation of Care Plan

1. Major anomalies
2. Respiratory distress

3. Apgar score of 5 at 5 minutes
4. Signs of sedation in the neonate
5. Maternal infection
   a. Increased temperature
   b. Greater than 24 hours since rupture of membranes
   c. Foul-smelling amniotic fluid
6. Severe hypertensive disease
7. Suspected intrauterine fetal growth retardation, or excessive size
8. Class A diabetes
9. Maternal drug addiction
10. Oligo-hydramnios or hydramnios
11. Prematurity, postmaturity, dysmaturity
12. Previous fetal wastage/neonatal death
13. No prenatal care

appendix

E

Prevention and Treatment of Ophthalmia Neonatorum*

Ophthalmia neonatorum (infectious conjunctivitis of the newborn) can be caused by a number of infectious agents. Approximately 100 years ago, Crede introduced the instillation of silver nitrate solution into the eyes of newborns. This prophylaxis has resulted in a marked reduction in the incidence of gonococcal ophthalmia neonatorum and ranks as one of the greatest preventive health accomplishments in ophthalmology. In 1973, a statement was prepared by the National Society to Prevent Blindness (NSPB) Committee on Ophthalmia Neonatorum. However, several factors dictate that the 1973 statement be updated, including inadequacies of silver nitrate prophylaxis; objections to the chemical conjunctivitis caused by silver nitrate; revised statements by other agencies; and new data on the incidence, clinical severity and etiologies of ophthalmia neonatorum.

The Committee on Ophthalmia Neonatorum of the National Society to Prevent Blindness makes the following recommendations on prophylaxis and treatment:

PREVENTION OF OPHTHALMIA NEONATORUM

The committee believes that the prevention of both gonococcal ophthalmia neonatorum, a potentially blinding disease, and chlamydial ophthalmia neonatorum, a common problem, must be considered.

RECOMMENDATIONS

1. Instillation of a prophylaxis agent in the eyes of all newborn infants.
2. Acceptable prophylactic agents which prevent gonococcal ophthalmia neonatorum include the following:
   a. Silver nitrate solution (1%) in single-dose ampules,

---

*A Statement by the National Society to Prevent Blindness Committee on Ophthalmia Neonatorum, 1981

    b. Erythromycin (0.5%) ophthalmic ointment or drops in single-use tubes or ampules,

    c. Tetracycline (1%) ophthalmic ointment or drops in single-use tubes or ampules.

3. Acceptable prophylactic agents which prevent chlamydial ophthalmia neonatorum include the following:

    a. Erythromycin (0.5%) ophthalmic ointment or drops in single-use tubes or ampules,

    b. Tetracycline (1%) ophthalmic ointment or drops in single-use tubes or ampules.

    Silver nitrate does not prevent chlamydial infections.

4. Prophylaxis agents should be given shortly after birth. A delay of up to one hour is probably acceptable and may facilitate initial maternal-infant bonding.

5. The importance of performing the instillation so the agent reaches all parts of the conjunctival surface is stressed. This can be accomplished by careful manipulation of the lids with fingers to insure spreading of the agent. If medication strikes only the eyelids and lid margins, but fails to reach the cornea, the instillation should be repeated. Prophylaxis should be applied as follows:

    a. Silver nitrate

        (1) Carefully clean eyelids and surrounding skin with sterile cotton, which may be moistened with sterile water.

        (2) Gently open baby's eyelids and instill two (2) drops of silver nitrate on the conjunctival sac. Allow the silver nitrate to run across the whole conjunctival sac. Carefully manipulate lids to insure spread of the drops. Repeat in the other eye. Use two (2) ampules, one for each eye.

        (3) After one minute, gently wipe excess silver nitrate from eyelids and surrounding skin with sterile water. Do not irrigate eyes.

    b. Ophthalmic ointment (erythromycin or tetracycline)

        (1) Carefully clean eyelids and surrounding skin with sterile cotton, which may be moistened with sterile water.

        (2) Gently open baby's eyelids and place a thin line of ointment, at least ½ inch (1–2 cm), along the junction of the bulbar and palpebral conjunctiva of the lower lid. Try to cover the whole lower conjunctival area. Carefully manipulate lids to insure spread of the ointment. Be careful not to touch the eyelid or eyeball with the tip of the tube. Repeat in other eye. Use one tube per baby.

        (3) After one minute, gently wipe excess ointment from eyelids and surrounding skin with sterile water. Do not irrigate eyes.

   c. Ophthalmic drops (erythromycin or tetracycline) Apply as silver nitrate.

6. The eye should not be irrigated after instillation of a prophylaxis agent. Irrigation may reduce the efficacy of prophylaxis and probably does not decrease the incidence of chemical conjunctivitis.

7. Infants born to mothers infected with agents which cause ophthalmia neonatorum may require special attention and systemic therapy, as well as prophylaxis. A single dose of aqueous crystalline penicillin G, 50,000 units/kg body weight for term and 20,000 units for low-birth-weight infants should be administered intravenously to infants born to mothers with gonorrhea.

8. The detection and appropriate treatment of infections in pregnant women, which may result in ophthalmia neonatorum, is encouraged.

9. All physicians and hospitals should be required to report cases of ophthalmia neonatorum and etiologic agent to state and local health departments so that incidence data may be obtained to determine the effectiveness of the control measures.

TREATMENT OF INFANTS WITH OPHTHALMIA NEONATORUM

Appropriate treatment should be utilized for all infants with ophthalmia neonatorum. Ophthalmologic consultation should be secured for such cases.

RECOMMENDATIONS

1. Specific infectious etiologic agents should be sought in each case.
2. Gonococcal ophthalmia neonatorum should be treated as follows:
   a. Infants should be hospitalized and isolated for 24 hours after initiation of treatment.
   b. Aqueous crystalline penicillin G, 50,000 units/kg body weight/day, in two doses intravenously, should be administered for seven (7) days.
   c. Saline irrigation of the eyes should be performed as often as needed.
   d. Topical antibiotics effective against gonococcus should be administered to prevent or treat early corneal involvement.

e. The emergence of pencillinase-producing *Neisseria gonorrhoeae* in the United States is recognized. The antibiotic susceptibility of gonococci causing ophthalmia neonatorum should be determined. If penicillin therapy fails, they should be treated with an aminoglycoside.

3. Chlamydial ophthalmia neonatorum should be treated with oral erythromycin, 30–50 mg/kg body weight/day, in four doses, for two weeks.

4. Herpetic conjunctivitis or keratitis, due to either type 1 or type 2 herpes simplex virus, may occur before overt signs of systemic disease develop. Such infants must be evaluated carefully. Topical treatment with trifluorothymidine five times daily until healed may be the best antiviral therapy in this setting.

5. Other bacterial causes of ophthalmia neonatorum can be adequately treated with either 0.5% erythromycin ointment or 10% sulfonamide ointment four times daily until resolution of the infection occurs.

6. Recurrent conjunctivitis may indicate that the nasolacrimal duct is not patent.

RESOURCES AND RECOMMENDED READING

Armstrong JR, Zacarias F, Rein MF: Ophthalmia neonatorum: A chart review. Pediatrics 57:884–892, 1976

Beem MO, Saxon EM: Respiratory tract colonization and distinctive pneumonia syndrome in infants infected with *Chlamydia trachomatis*. N Engl J Med 296:306–310, 1977

Brook I, Martin WJ, Finegold SM: Effect of silver nitrate application on the conjunctival flora of the newborn and the occurrence of clostridial conjunctivitis. J Pediatr Ophthalmol Strabismus 15:179–183, 1978

Burns RP, Rhodes DH: *Pseudomonas* eye infection as a cause of death in premature infants. Arch Ophthalmol 65:517–527, 1961

Chandler JW, Alexander ER, et al: Ophthalmia neonatorum associated with maternal chlamydial infections. Trans Am Acad Ophthalmol Otolaryngol 83:302–308, 1977

Cohen KL, McCarthy LR: *Haemophilus influenzae* ophthalmia neonatorum. Arch Ophthalmol 98:1214–1215, 1980

Goscienski PJ, Sexton RR: Follow-up studies in neonatal inclusion conjunctivitis. Am J Dis Child 124:180–182, 1972

Grayston JT, Wang SP: New knowledge of *Chlamydia* and the diseases they cause. J Infect Dis 132:87–105, 1975

Hagler WS, Walters PV, Nahmias AJ: Ocular involvement in neonatal herpes simplex virus infection. Arch Ophthalmol 82:169–176, 1969

Hammerschlag MR, Chandler JW, Alexander ER, et al: Erythromycin ointment for ocular prophylaxis of neonatal chlamydial infection. JAMA 244:2291–2293, 1980

Hansen T, Burns RP, Allen A: Gonorrheal conjunctivitis: An old disease returned. JAMA 195:1156, 1966

Hansman D: Neonatal meningococcal conjunctivitis. Br Med J 1:748, 1972

Harrison HR, English MG, Lee CK, et al: *Chlamydia trachomatis* infant pneumonitis. N Engl J Med 298:702–708, 1978

Kaivonen M: Prophylaxis of ophthalmia neonatorum. Acta Ophthalmologica [Suppl] 79:7–70, 1965

McCracken GH, Eichenwald HF: Antimicrobial therapy in infants and children. Part II. Review of antimicrobial agents. J Pediatr 93:357–377, 1978

Morhorst CH, Dawson CR: Sequalae of neonatal inclusion conjunctivitis and associated disease in parents. Am J Ophthalmol 71:861–867, 1971

Nahmias AJ, Visintine AM, Caldwell DR, et al: Eye infections with herpes simplex viruses in neonates. Surv Ophthalmol 21:100–105, 1976

Nishida H, Risenberg HM: Silver nitrate ophthalmic solution and chemical conjunctivitis. Pediatrics 56:368–373, 1975

Ostler HB: Oculogenital disease. Surv Ophthalmol 20:233–246, 1976

Prentice JF, Hutchinson GR, Taylor-Robinson D: A microbiological study of neonatal conjunctivae and conjunctivitis. Br J Ophthalmol 61:601–607, 1977

Rothenberg R: Ophthalmia neonatorum due to *Neisseria gonorrhoeae:* Prevention and treatment. Sex Transm Dis [Suppl] 6:187–191, 1979

Rowe DS, Aicardi EZ, Dawson CR, et al: Purulent ocular discharge in neonates: Significance of *Chlaymdia trachomatis.* Pediatrics 63:628–632, 1979

Schacter J, Holt J, Goodner E, et al: Prospective study of chlamydial infection in neonates. Lancet 2:377–380, 1979

Schacter J: Chlamydial infections (3 reports). N Engl J Med 298:428–435, 540–549, 1978

Thygeson P: Historical review of oculogenital disease. Am J Ophthalmol 71:975–985, 1971

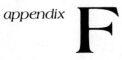

Maternal Consultation/ Transfer Record

Date of referral call _____ Time _____
Person receiving call _____
Patient's _____
Referring physician _____
Primary physician _____
Referring hospital _____
Person calling _____
Reason for admission _____
_____

Maternal History

1. Age _____
2. Gravida _____
3. Para _____
4. Abortion _____
5. Weeks of gestation _____
6. Last menstrual period _____ Estimated date of confinement _____

7. Onset of contractions _____
8. Frequency of contractions _____
9. Cervical dilation _____
10. Evidence of vaginal bleeding _____
11. Rupture of membranes? Yes _____ No _____ Time _____
12. Fetal heart rate: Infant 1 _____ Infant 2 _____ Other _____
13. a. Temperature _____ b. Blood pressure _____ c. Pulse _____

14. Blood type _____
15. Referral history _____
    Relevant health problems _____
    _____

    Perinatal history _____
    _____

    Reason for transfer _____
    _____

16. Referral plan _____
    _____

17. Transported by _____
    _____

18. Assessment by _____
    Date _____

G

Newborn Consultation/ Transfer Record

DATE OF REF. CALL: _ / _ / _

TIME CALL RECEIVED _____

PERSON RECEIVING CALL

SEX (circle one):
1. female
2. male
3. other

PATIENT IDENTIFICATION

INFANT'S LAST NAME   FIRST NAME

INSURANCE

REFERRING MD NAME   ( )   PHONE

MD WHO DELIVERED INFANT ("X" over Dr. if not appropriate)   ( )   PHONE

PRIMARY MD NAME   ( )   PHONE

HOSPITAL DELIVERED AT   DELIV. CITY, STATE   ZIP

REFERRING HOSPITAL NAME   CITY, STATE   ZIP

BIRTHDATE: _ / _ / _   BIRTHWT.: _ _ _ _ gm   EGA: _ _

NAME OF PERSON CALLING   ( )   REF. HOSP. PHONE

REF. APGARS
1 min
5 min

MATERNAL HISTORY:
1. Age: _ _
2. Grav: _ _
3. Para: _ _
4. Abo: _ _

OTHER SIGNIFICANT INFORMATION

REFERRAL HISTORY (incl. lab & x-ray results):

PRELIMINARY DIAGNOSIS:

OXYGEN DELIVERY:	VENT	MODE/BLOOD	Gas	Site
1. Nasotrach	Time			
2. Orotrach	CPAP			
3. Nasal prongs	PIP			
4. Mask	PEEP			
5. Tracheostomy	Rate			
6. Nasopharyngeal	IT			
8. Other	FiO_2			
9. Unknown	Po_2			
0. None	Pco_2			
	pH			
VENT MODE:	BE			
1. Bagging	Site			
2. Respirator				
8. Other				
9. Unknown				
0. None				

FLUID LINES PLACED? (Circle all that apply.)

	Solution	Rate
1. Peripheral		
2. U/A		
3. U/V		
4. Other (specify)		
5. None		

REF TEMP: _ _ °C
REF DEXTROSTIX: _ _ MG%
REF GLUCOSE: _ _ MG%
REF HCT: _ _ %
REF BLOOD PRESSURE: _ _ / _ _

	Yes	No
1. Apnea?	_	_
2. X-rays taken?	_	_
3. Blood cultures?	_	_
4. Antibiotics given?	_	_
5. OG tube?	_	_

HOUSE OFFICER ASSESSMENT AND INSTRUCTIONS:

	Yes	No
1. Temp adequate?	_	_
2. Monitoring adeq?	_	_
3. Blood volume adequate?	_	_
4. Glucose adequate?	_	_
5. Ventilation adequate?	_	_
6. Sepsis suspected?	_	_
7. Meds appropriate?	_	_
8. Other (instructions):		

RECOMMENDATIONS:

TYPE OF REFERRAL

DATE _____

ASSESSMENT BY (last name only)

ATTENDING CONSULTANT (last name only)

H

Equipment and Medication for Maternal-Neonatal Transport

I. Maternal
  A. Adult resuscitation equipment
    1. Airways
       1 each #'s 4, 3, 2, 1, 0,
         neonate
       1 epistix
    2. Intubation
       1 bottle xylocaine viscous
       1 laryngoscope handle
       1 each Miller blades #'s 1,
         2; Foregger #'s 1, 3, 4
       1 hemostat
       2 McGill forceps; 1 small,
         1 large

       1 each ET tubes #'s 2.5,
         3.0, 3.5, 4.0, 4.5, 5.0,
         5.5, 6.0, 6.5, 7.0, 7.5, 8.0
       3 10-cc syringes
       3 stylets; 1 small, 2 large

    3. Chest aspiration set
       1 50-cc syringe
       1 3-way stopcock
       1 tourniquet connecting
         tube

       1 angiocath, #14
       1 Heimlich valve

    4. IV equipment
       1 tourniquet
       1 plastic tape
       1 adhesive tape, alcohol
         wipes, Bandaids
       1 each intracath; small,
         medium, large
       1 each angiocath #'s 22,
         20, 18, 14

       2 size #16 angiocath
       2 500-cc LR with regular
         IV tubing
       1 250-cc D_5W with
         pediatric IV tubing

    5. Other
       BP Cuff

B. Adult resuscitation drugs
   1. Narcotics
      1 case sealed with wire
         split shot
      1 tubex holder
      2 tubex benadryl 50 mg

      2 tubex morphine sulfate
         10 mg
      2 tubex morphine sulfate
         15 mg
      2 tubex phenobarbital 2 g

   2. Other drugs
      2 ampules aminophylline
         500 mg
      2 ammonia inhalants
         anectine (sucostrin) in
         refrigerator
      3 ampules antilirium
         (physostigmine)
      1 ampule aqua mephyton
         10 mg
      1 vial aramine 10 cc
      4 atropine bristoject 1 mg
      1 vial atropine multidose
         vial
      1 water 30 cc
      1 NaCL 30 cc
      1 ampule calcium chloride
         10 cc (1 g)
      1 vial decadron multidose
      2 dextrose 50% bristoject
         50 cc
      2 ampules digoxin 0.5 mg
      2 ampules dramamine 1
         cc (50 mg/cc)
      1 dramamine 50 mg 12/
         pack (oral)
      4 ampules epinephrine
         1:1000 (1 mg)

      4 epinephrine bristoject
         1:10,000 (1 mg)
      1 vial glucagon
      2 ipecac syrup
      2 ampules isuprel 0.5 mg
      4 isuprel bristoject 1 mg
      1 lacril (artificial tears)
      4 ampules lasix 20 mg
      2 ampules levophed 4 cc
      2 lidocaine addajet 1 g
      4 lidocaine bristoject 100
         mg methergine 1 cc (in
         refrigerator)
     10 ampules narcan 0.4 mg
      1 vial potassium chloride
         40 mEq
      1 vial protopam
      6 sodium bicarbonate
         bristoject 44.6 mEq
      1 vial solu cortef 1 g
      1 vial solu medrol 1 g
      3 Valium 10 mg
      1 vial xylocaine 1%
      1 NaCL 100 mEq/40 cc
      4 ampules $MgSO_4$ 10%—
         10 cc

3. Top of case

   alcohol swabs

   2 each blood tubes; red,
     lavender and green tops

   5 each syringes; 3, 5, 10
     cc, TB and insulin

   5 each needles #'s 15,19,
     20, 21, 23, 25 gauge

   1 each 60-cc needle tip
     syringe

   1 each Toomey syringe

   2 each vacutainer holders
     and needles

C. Obstetric delivery equipment (OB case)

  1. Top

    4 pair gloves; 2 #7, 1
      #7½, 1 #8

    2 10/pkg. 4 × 4's

    1 bulb syringe

    2 silver swaddlers

    2 DeLee suctions

    3 neonate electrodes

    1 plastic bag

    2 disp. scalpels

    2 pediatric drips

  2. Pocket

    2 thermometers

    2 scalp vein 25 gauge

    several packages surgilube

    pHisoHex

    several Alco wipes

    2 cord clamps

    2 chromic suture (3–0)

    1 Y connector

  3. Bottom

    3 chux

    2 sterile drapes

    2 polylined towels

    2 sterile green towels

    2 OB pads, sterile

    2 razors

    1 dextrostix with
      Bandaids and lancets

    1 fetoscope

    1 Doppler

    several needles

    2 scissors (one with long
      handles)

    1 needle holder

    1 pick-up forcep

    4 exam gloves, large,
      single, sterile

    2 Kling 2"

    1 hemostat

  4. Drugs

    1 30 cc 1% lidocaine

    5 $MgSO_4$ 50%

    2 $MgSO_4$ 10%

    2 apresoline 20 mg/cc

    3 1-cc ampule syntocin (10
      units)

    1000 cc 10% alcohol in
      5% dextrose

II. Neonatal

A. Essential equipment

Transport incubator	Thermometer
Oxygen supply (including delivery tubing flowmeter and humidifier)	Stethoscope
	Heart rate monitor
	Blood pressure unit
Compressed air	Emergency drugs
Oxygen analyzer	Intraveneous set-up and
Oxygen hood	solutions (plastic bottles
Ventilation bag and mask	ideal for IV solutions)
Endotracheal tubes	Constant infusion pump
(appropriate sizes)	Thoracocentesis set
Laryngoscope	Dextrostix
Suction apparatus	

Optional but desirable

Radiant heat shield	Transcutaneous O_2
Silver swaddler	monitor
Chemical warming mattress	Direct line arterial
Electronic thermometer	pressure monitor
Oxygen/air blender	Umbilical catheterization
Constant positive airway	tray
pressure unit	Thoracostomy tray
Mechanical ventilator	Heimlich valves
(capable of running off compressed gas)	

B. Neonatal transport kit equipment and medications inventory

Top shelf

1 laryngoscope	2 face masks (sizes 1 and 0)
2 laryngoscope blades (Miller 0, Miller 1)	NT Tubes (2.5, 3.0, 3.5, 4.0) 2 each
1 spare laryngoscope bulb (small size)	1 Magill forceps
	4 gauze swabs (2 by 2)
2 spare laryngoscope batteries (size AA)	3 needle electrodes
	6 chest electrodes
1 packet sterile lubricant	1 stylet
1 portawarm crystals	1 tank key
1 scissors	3 heart monitor lead wires
1 anesthesia bag	Locker combination

Second shelf

6 thermometers
2 feeding tubes (8 Fr)
2 stopcock plugs
2 3-way stopcocks
3 Christmas trees
8 needles (2 each of 18, 20, 22, 25 gauge)
Saran wrap
4 limb restraints
Safety pins
Rubber bands
Alcohol swabs
3 corks
Cotton balls
Betadine swabs

Third shelf

3 tuberculin syringes with needles
6 3-cc syringes (2 each with 20, 22, 25 gauge needles)
2 12-cc syringes
2 20-cc syringes
5 scalp vein needles (3 each of 25 gauge; 1 each of 21, 23, 27 gauge)
2 rolls adhesive tape (½ and 1 inch)
1 roll paper tape (1 inch)
2 rolls dermiclear tape (½ inch)
3 Q-tips
1 wooden tongue blade
2 paper tape measure
1 disposable razor
4 plastic medicine cups (IV caps)

2 sutures with curved needles (4–0)
8 Bandaids
5 lancets
1 bottle capillary tubes
1 bottle dextrostix reagent strips
1 bottle Tincture benzoin
1 bottle alcohol
1 bottle betadine
1 pacifier
1 umbilical tape
1 yellow top tube
3 blunt adapters, 1 each 17, 19, 20 gauge

1 arm board
2 22-gauge quik caths and 1 27-gauge quik cath
3 IV "Medication Added" Labels
Drugs:
Heparin 1000 u/ml
Saline (10-ml vial)
Sterile H_2O (10-ml vial)
Flush solv D5 ¼ NS = 2 u Heparin/cc
NaCL 2.5 mEq/cc (30 cc)
KAc 2 mEq/1 cc (30 cc)
$NaHCO_3$ 8.4% (30 cc)
Ampicillin 250-mg vial
Gentamicin 2-cc vial (10 mg/cc)
Aspirin and dramamine

Bottom shelf

4 suction catheters and glove pack; 1 5/6 Fr, 2 8 Fr, 1 10 Fr

1 Milli-pore filter

1 12 Fr sump tube

4 sterile glove packs (1 each of sizes 6, 6½, 7, 7½)

1 Metriset

1 pediatric IV set

1 500-ml bag $D_{10}W$

1 extension tubing (20 inch)

1 stethoscope

4 arterial catheters (2 each of 3½, 5 Fr)

2 Heimlich set-ups:
    2 Heimlich valves
    2 16-g medicuts
    2 stopcocks (3-way)
    2 extension tubing (for attachment to Medicut)
    2 green heimlich valve adaptors

1 medication kit containing
    2 NAHCO₃ 4.2% (10-ml syringes)

Aquamephyton (pediatric); 2 phenobarbital; 5% albumin; calcium gluconate; 2 narcan; digoxin (pediatric); lasix; decadron; epinephrine (10-ml syringe); lidocaine; isuprel; dopamine; prisocline

$D_{50}W$; dilantin; 2 glass filters

(See medications list for quantities and preparation strengths.)

2 thoracocentesis set-ups:
    2 60-cc syringes
    2 3-way stopcocks
    2 23-g butterflies

1 DeLee suction with mucus trap

4 Holter pump tubings (2 size A, 2 size C)

1 silver swaddler

1 bowel bag

1 red rubber catheter (10 Fr)

1 Sphygmomanometer with 2 cuffs (infant and newborn)

Jelly for BP transducer

2 24-hour urine bags, 1 newborn, 1 pediatric

4 trocar cannulas (2 10 Fr, 2 12 Fr)

2 blood culture bottles

1 steridrape

1 T-connector

1 platelet infusion set

1 blood filter

Mini UA/thoracotomy set
1. Sterile drapes, 2
2. Iris forceps
3. Needle holder
4. Scissor
5. Curved forceps, 2
6. Tongue tissue forcep
7. Sterile 2 × 2
8. Cath adaptor
9. Umbilical tape
10. Scalpel and blade

appendix **I.**

Adoption Communication Sheet

Form completed by _____
Name   Date   /   Time

Amended by _____
Name   Date   /   Time

Amended by _____
Name   Date   /   Time

Patient is on "No Information."
Social Service Department has been notified of this pending adoption.

Per previous communication, Mother wishes:

- ☐ To see infant
- ☐ To know sex of infant
- ☐ To be on OB floor
- ☐ No persons other than Mother to see infant
- ☐ Persons other than Mother to see infant as indicated below:

- ☐ Not to see infant
- ☐ Not to know sex of infant
- ☐ To be off OB floor

_____

Agency Adoption: ☐ *Private Adoption:*

Caseworker _____   Attorney _____

Agency _____   Phone No. _____

Phone No. _____ Work _____ Home _____

Adoptive family may see infant per arrangement below: _____

_____

_____

_____

_____

Physician's comments: _____

_____

_____
Signature

Discharge:

Released by _____ Picked up by _____ Date __/__ Time

INDEX

Abnormalities, congenital, 235–236
Abortion, definition of, 200
Acidosis, neonatal, 71
Acoustic characteristics in pediatric
    unit, 35
Admission/observation areas
    in obstetric unit, 16
    in pediatric unit, 26
Admission procedure, in labor and
    delivery area, 59–60
Adoption, 237–240
    adoptive parents in, 240
    birth mother in, 239–240
    communication sheet used in, 275
    legal aspects of, 238
    and nursery observations, 238–
        239
    physical evaluation in, 239
    procedures in, 237–239
Advisory group for perinatal care, 8
Age
    conceptional, definition of, 202
    gestational. *See* Gestational age
Aircraft, for transport of patients,
    192
Alternative birth centers,
    freestanding, 58–59
Ambulances, for transport of
    patients, 192
Ambulation, postpartum, 75
Amniocentesis, 209
Amniotomy, in labor, induction, 65
Analgesia, in labor and delivery, 61
Anesthesia, in labor and delivery,
    61–62
Antenatal detection of genetic
    disorders, 207–211
    amniocentesis in, 209

fetoscopy in, 209–210
and identification of risk factors,
    207–209
indications for, 210–211
laboratory studies in, 210
Antepartum care, 48–58
    education programs in, 56–58
    and establishment of expected
        date of confinement, 50
    follow-up visits in, 52
    history-taking in, 49–50
    immunizations in, 143–144, 145
    laboratory tests in, 51
    nutrition in. *See* Nutrition
    physical examination in, 50
    and preconceptional counseling,
        257–259
    psychosocial support in, 58
    in pyelonephritis, 143
    risk assessment in, 8–9, 52–56
    rubella prevention and
        management in, 133–134
    serial surveillance in, 48–56
Antibiotics
    for neonates, 119
    prophylactic, for obstetric
        patients, 116–117
    with lactation, 123
Antiseptics
    for disinfection of equipment, 156
    for hand-washing, 112
    for skin care in newborn, 120
Apgar scores, 68–69
Assessment. *See* Evaluation

Bacterial colonization of neonates,
    107–108